R6/3

ECZEMA AND DERMATITIS

Rona MacKie is Professor of Dermatology at the University of Glasgow in Scotland. She has twenty years specialized clinical experience of treating skin disease.

She is a member of the European Society of Dermatological Research and has written numerous scientific papers as well as a specialist textbook of dermatology.

Prof MacKie is married with two children and lives in Glasgow.

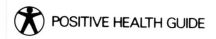

POSITIVE HEALTH GUIDE

ECZEMA
AND
DERMATITIS

How to cope
with inflamed skin

Prof Rona MacKie,
MD, FRCP

MARTIN DUNITZ

© Rona MacKie 1983

First published in the United Kingdom in 1983
by Martin Dunitz Ltd, London

British Library Cataloguing-in-Publication Data
MacKie, Rona M.
   Eczema and dermatitis.–(Positive health guide)
   1. Dermatology
   I. Title   II. Series
   616.5   RL71
ISBN 0–906348–42–0
ISBN 0–906348–41–2 Pbk

Phototypeset in Garamond by Input
Typesetting Ltd, London

Printed in Singapore

CONTENTS

INTRODUCTION

My aim in writing this book is to bring to the attention of as many people as possible the problems connected with dermatitis or eczema. In particular, I want to offer some practical advice to those of you who suffer from the disease as well as to those who are parents of children with the problem.

But first, a word about the names used to describe this common skin disease. For many the words 'eczema' and 'dermatitis' create confusion. Some people explain the use of two words to describe what looks like the same disease by calling the skin eruptions that are caused by handling various substances 'dermatitis', and the more severe and chronic condition 'eczema'.

In fact, neither is true. The word eczema means literally 'boiling out' in the original Greek and was at one time used to describe red, irritable, sore and itching skin due to internal causes, whereas dermatitis – which means inflammation of the skin – was used to describe the same sort of picture due to external sources. Nowadays, though, the idea of dividing skin conditions in this way is recognized as being too simple and the majority of skin specialists consider that the words mean the same thing.

Like many of my colleagues in the medical profession, I have a personal preference for the word 'dermatitis', and I have used this throughout the text – but remember that whichever term is used the other could equally well be substituted.

To anyone with dermatitis it seems that the rest of the population can be divided into two classes – those who treat any skin blemishes as something contagious, and to be shunned and (a much smaller class) those who think the problem is a relatively trivial one. To those who suffer from the problem neither attitude is in the least helpful. We can help disguise the rashes where that's possible and prescribe treatment to heal and to counter the overwhelming desire to scratch. The other problem, however, is the psychological one – the blow to one's confidence, the feeling of isolation, of being 'different' – that can develop, particularly in someone who has had the disease since childhood. I hope that all who come into contact with those who suffer from dermatitis – their families, friends, teachers and colleagues – may gain new insights into the problem through reading this book and offer their confidence, support and affection.

Accurate figures for the number of people suffering from dermatitis are difficult to obtain. Many sufferers do not seek medical help at all, others are seen by their family doctor. As survey figures are usually taken only from hospital records, many cases are missed. However, even though usually only the most severe cases are referred to a skin specialist, or dermatologist, they still make up a large part – one-third of all those attending – of the specialist's workload. Indeed, dermatitis forms part of a trio – with acne and psoriasis – of the commonest skin problems today.

An important point to remember is that most people with dermatitis have only very mild forms of the disease, and that the risk of some of the more severe or worrying complications described in certain sections of the book is very small. At the same time I should emphasize also that many forms of dermatitis are very common, particularly in young children, and so some understanding of the disease will make it easier for parents and for sufferers to cope with the condition in terms of their general health as well as in their work and leisure activities. As research into the causes of dermatitis gathers momentum, we can look forward to new treatments, better prevention methods – and perhaps even a cure.

In the treatment of dermatitis as in other branches of medicine, there are areas in which doctors 'agree to disagree'. No one point of view is right, another wrong. What is right at one time in the treatment of a disease is often quite wrong at another. The use of mild steroid creams, for example, is the right treatment 90 per cent of the time for someone with dermatitis, but becomes wrong if they develop a virus infection as well. One or two of you may find apparent differences between my approach to treatment and that prescribed by your own doctor. In that case, you should consult him or her and take the advice offered. No one knows your own case better than the medical practitioner with whom you are regularly in contact.

Finally, a word about facts and figures: you will find scattered throughout the book reference to numbers of people who suffer from a certain type of dermatitis, or numbers of people who have certain diseases. These figures vary throughout the world and will be different, for example, in an industrial city and a country town. So remember, they are only a rough guide.

Drug names

Throughout the book drugs are referred to only by their British trade names. Where appropriate, their American, Canadian, Australian and South African equivalents are listed in the International Drug Name Equivalents section at the end of the book.

1 WHAT IS DERMATITIS?

Normal healthy skin is something most of us take for granted – we only appreciate how good it is to have it there protecting us when it goes wrong. It is only when we cut ourselves, or get sunburn, that the pain, or the peeling and itch make us uncomfortably aware of our skin, but as this heals we once again forget about it.

For the person with dermatitis this marvellous normality cannot be taken for granted – his or her skin is sensitive, itchy and sore, sometimes distressingly so. For those who are severely affected, it can interfere with friendships, schoolwork, occupations, even sports and hobbies – their whole lives, in fact. So, what is it that goes wrong with our skin and causes dermatitis? Why does it affect some people and not others? As we progress through the book the answers will become clear. Meanwhile, we should perhaps take a look at our skin and the way it works and come to know some of the terms we shall be meeting.

The skin, a vital organ

Our skin is made up of two main parts. There is a thick, elastic lower layer, the dermis, which contains a network of fine blood vessels (capillaries); the nerves that supply sensation to the skin; both sebaceous – or grease-secreting – and sweat glands; and the tough fibres called collagen, and the elastic fibres that give our skin its suppleness. Fine body hairs also grow from the dermis.

Above the dermis is a thin firm outer layer, the epidermis, at the base of which new cells are formed so that the older ones are being continually pushed to the surface and shed. As these epidermal cells travel to the surface they change their shape and structure and by the time they reach the outermost scaly layer of our skin they are composed almost entirely of a material called keratin, which also forms our hair and nails.

The variety of tiny glands contained in our skin secretes different materials. The entire body surface has a very rich supply of sweat

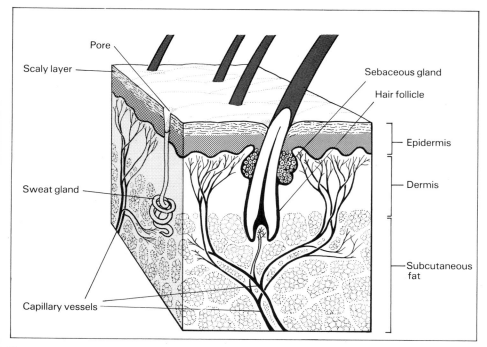

The main features of normal skin.

glands that continually allow evaporation of moisture from the skin surface. A second form of sweat gland is mainly found in larger numbers in the armpit, which becomes stimulated into activity by stress or tension. The third type of gland is quite different and is usually associated with the roots of the fine hairs that cover most of our body. These are the sebaceous glands which secrete sebum, a greasy material. They are very small in childhood and become functional only at puberty when they may become temporarily overactive and cause acne, an extremely common problem among teenagers. The sebaceous glands are found in larger numbers on the skin of the face, the scalp, the upper chest and the back.

Our skin is therefore very much more than just an outer cover — it is an important organ and vital to health and life. Healthy normal skin has several important functions including:

1. Regulating body temperature by giving off heat from the many small vessels in the skin and through the evaporation of sweat.

2. Getting rid of some waste products.

3. Being an organ of touch and making us aware of our environment.

4. Keeping out infection-causing bacteria, which cannot digest the dried scales at the surface and make their way through them.

5. Helping to protect the body from being burnt by the sun, through the production of pigment.

6. Manufacturing some of our quota of vitamin D, needed by the body to help build the tissues of our bones.

All of these functions could be partly impaired through various skin diseases.

What happens to your skin when you get dermatitis?

When we look through the microscope at the skin of someone with dermatitis, we notice in the epidermis and dermis a large number of cells that are normally found mainly in the blood. These are white blood cells that release tiny quantities of substances which irritate the skin cells and set up a cycle of irritation, itch and redness, leading to scratching, more irritation, swelling and redness. If this inflammation is not treated successfully, or if it is repeatedly scratched and the surface of the skin is broken, then the condition becomes chronic. One consolation to dermatitis sufferers is that once cleared up, it doesn't leave scars.

The three stages

Although there are many types of dermatitis, and I shall be describing them later in the chapter, they all follow a more or less well-defined pattern. Of course, treatment or natural improvement often means that the disease doesn't progress beyond the first or second stage. However, the pattern that the various forms of dermatitis will follow if left untreated falls into three stages, depending on the length of time the skin has been irritated.

1. Acute   In this stage the skin is red, inflamed, moist and swollen, and will feel both itchy and painful. Often, tiny blisters appear which eventually burst and weep. The acute stage, as its name suggests, is painful, but fortunately it is also short-lived.

2. Subacute   This stage is not so severe, but it does last longer than

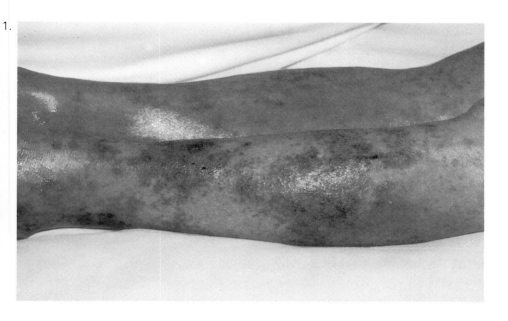

1. The painful, inflamed acute stage. 2. A crust may form during the subacute stage.
3. The long-term chronic stage when the skin thickens and becomes scaly.

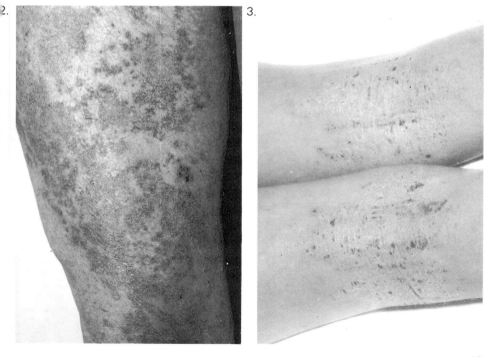

the acute stage. Now the moisture and swelling of the skin dies down a little and a crust may form, but redness, scaling and itch are all still troublesome.

Itchiness causes scratching, particularly in young children, and once the skin has been broken infection very quickly develops. The infection will bring with it pain, throbbing and collections of white blood cells (pus) around the wounded areas – all indications of the subacute stage.

If the infection is severe it may spread from the actual site of the dermatitis. If the dermatitis was on the hands, for example, you may be able to see the infection spreading as thin red lines travelling up the arm, particularly on the inside of the arm. When the infection reaches the protective lymph glands under the arm they may become enlarged and tender.

3. Chronic   In this long-term phase of dermatitis the main problem is itch, which leads to scratching or rubbing. This in turn causes thickening of the skin of the affected area which shows up as a raised scaly patch with the normal skin lines showing up in an exaggerated pattern. This thickening (known as lichenification) is a defence mechanism on the part of the body in an effort to prevent damage to the skin by further scratching, and can clear dramatically if the scratching or rubbing is stopped. There have been cases where a sufferer from chronic dermatitis has broken a limb on which these thickened patches are present. After the limb has been encased in plaster-of-Paris for a short period, the patches on the protected area melt away with surprising speed.

Now it is quite possible to have all these stages or 'ages' of dermatitis present at the same time. For instance you may have a child with an acute and perhaps infected atopic dermatitis on his cheeks, subacute areas that have been scratched and infected on his hands, and chronic patches of thickened lined skin behind his knees.

What kinds of dermatitis are there?

Although many types of dermatitis look alike, and may follow the same pattern of severity, there are several different varieties of the disease. Eight of the commoner types are listed below, but even this is not the complete catalogue.

1. Atopic dermatitis (childhood eczema)

2. Contact dermatitis
3. Varicose (or stasis) dermatitis
4. Seborrhoeic dermatitis
5. Napkin dermatitis (nappy or diaper rash)
6. Neurodermatitis ('nervous' dermatitis)
7. Nummular (discoid or coin-shaped) dermatitis
8. Exfoliative (severely scaling) dermatitis.

The body site involved may give a clue to the doctor as to which type of dermatitis is present. For example, problems on the skin of a child's face, the front of the elbows and behind the knees all suggest atopic dermatitis, whereas a dermatitis rash on the legs over varicose veins in an older person suggests stasis, or varicose, dermatitis.

Atopic dermatitis (childhood eczema)

This is the commonest form of dermatitis. It tends to run in families and can be inherited from either the mother's or the father's side of the family. It can also develop in a child with no family history of

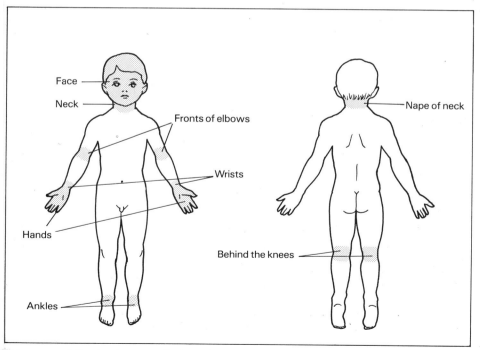

The areas of the body most likely to be affected by atopic dermatitis (also known as childhood eczema).

the disease. As many as one family in ten may have past or present members affected with this condition. Although the great majority of cases occur in infancy and childhood (see chapter two), atopic dermatitis can develop at any time throughout life, but it is very rare indeed in the elderly. It affects roughly equal numbers of girls and boys.

It usually begins with patches of itching, dry irritable skin on the face, behind the ears and knees and in the skin folds of the elbows and neck. Young children find it impossible not to scratch these areas, which usually means that they become open and infected.

Atopic dermatitis is known to occur frequently in people who also have asthma and hay fever, or in people whose families have someone with asthma or hay fever – a brother or sister perhaps. Another pattern is that someone may have attacks of dermatitis that alternate with attacks of asthma with the skin being 'active' when the asthma is 'quiet', and vice versa.

Contact dermatitis

This is caused, as the name suggests, by direct contact with some substance or material that sets up a reaction in or on the skin. As I shall be showing in chapter three, there is a large number of substances that can trigger off the condition; but contact dermatitis can be divided largely into two very distinct types:

1. Irritant contact dermatitis   In this type, which affects around 5 per cent of the population, the substance causing the problem gives rise to red irritant patches of dermatitis on anyone whose skin comes into contact with the material. You will start to have trouble with your skin the first time you handle the material. It usually takes the form of redness and itch on whichever part of the skin touches the material.

2. Allergic, or sensitization, contact dermatitis   In this type the substance causing the dermatitis can be handled without any ill-effect by most of us and only an unfortunate minority who touch it develop dermatitis. If you are one of this minority you will have come into contact with this particular material at some time in the past, and as a result of this contact a group of white blood cells, known as the T lymphocytes, develop a particular recognition or 'memory' for the material. When you next touch the material these specialist cells multiply rapidly and trigger off the dermatitis reaction. You may not be able to pin-point the cause straight away because there may be

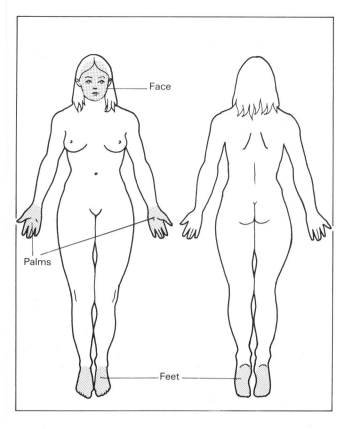

The areas of the body most often affected by contact dermatitis.

quite a long interval of perhaps from four to seven days between handling the material and developing a rash. What is more, the rash may develop on parts of your body some distance from where you actually touched the material, thus confusing everyone. Another difficulty is that it is possible to handle a material for many years without any problems, and then suddenly, for no known reason, to develop a sensitivity to this material.

Varicose (or stasis) dermatitis

This is the term used to describe the fragile reddish skin that develops around the ankles of many people who suffer from varicose veins (see chapter three). This type of dermatitis is very common in those who have had untreated varicose veins for a long time.

The sluggish blood flow through these veins means that the skin and tissues of the ankles are poorly nourished and frequently become irritable and itchy. You may find that your ankles take on a speckled appearance. This is due to small blood vessels bursting, and leaking

17

into the skin. The overlying outer layer of skin, the epidermis, becomes very thin and delicate and is easily broken, so if you do have these symptoms be especially careful not to knock your legs or ankles on furniture and do not scratch the area.

Once broken, this skin is very slow to heal and the final result of this form of dermatitis may be a varicose ulcer. These ulcers are very difficult to heal, and have an unhappy habit of breaking down again. The important point here is to seek early treatment for your varicose veins before this type of skin problem arises. This is a situation where prevention is very much better than cure.

Seborrhoeic dermatitis
There are two distinct forms of this condition, infantile and adult seborrhoeic dermatitis. At the present time there is no evidence despite the shared name to suggest that the two are in any way related, except that the areas affected are those where sebaceous glands are most numerous.

1. Infantile As its name suggests, this type is seen only in babies. The baby usually has a greasy, scaly, 'scurfy' scalp (known as 'cradle cap'), and redness and scaling in the body folds. In spite of what may look like a sore and irritable skin, the child is cheerful, and eats and sleeps well. It's a good example of a condition that upsets you more than your child. The problem usually arises in the first three months of a baby's life and clears by the time the child is between six and nine months old. (See chapter two.)

2. Adult This is a more chronic problem that tends to affect men more often than women (see chapter three). Pink scaly patches develop on the scalp, the face, the front of the chest and in the body folds. The condition tends to be aggravated by a hot humid climate, and is also irritated by creams and ointments. A problem that often precedes this condition is severe dandruff, and a persistently itchy scalp.

Adult seborrhoeic dermatitis used to be very common before 1940, and then, for reasons we don't yet understand, all but disappeared for the next twenty years. In the 1970s and '80s it has again become more prevalent.

Napkin dermatitis (nappy or diaper rash)
This is a common form of dermatitis in babies (see chapter two) and results from the baby's skin being in contact with a damp napkin,

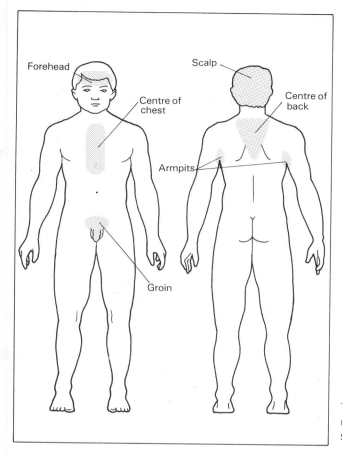

The areas of the body usually affected by adult seborrhoeic dermatitis.

or diaper. It doesn't seem to make any difference whether the nappies are the disposable type or made of Terry towelling or muslin. The use of waterproof plastic or rubber pants will increase the likelihood of this kind of dermatitis as more moisture is retained to irritate the skin.

You will find that your child's buttocks become red and possibly moist, but that the skin in the body folds, particularly at the front of the groin area, are relatively free of problems. An infection often associated with this condition is caused by a yeast fungus (candida) which can be recognized by the red circular patches around the edges of the main central area of irritation. These are called 'satellite lesions'.

This common form of dermatitis clears quickly if the child's skin is kept clean and dry and is not usually associated with the more severe forms of dermatitis.

The following three types of dermatitis are much rarer than the ones already described, and your chances of getting them are very slim.

Neurodermatitis ('nervous' dermatitis)

You may be one of a small number of people who develop a small, extremely itchy patch of skin. Persistent scratching of this patch (it's often on the arms or the back of the neck) gives rise to a circular, raised, thickened area of skin. Before you realize it, the scratching has become a habit. It is particularly noticeable when you are tired or tense, and as the scratching provokes a vicious circle of itch/scratch/itch it can be extremely difficult to break. 'Nervous' dermatitis can be exceptionally itchy and uncomfortable despite the small size of the patch of skin involved (see chapter seven).

Nummular (discoid or coin-shaped) dermatitis

The name describes the appearance of small circular patches of dermatitis. They appear most often on arms and legs and occur in both young adults and older people. It may occur in people who had atopic dermatitis when they were young. These patches have a tendency to become infected and may get very much worse at times of stress, worry, and increased tension (see chapter seven).

Exfoliative (severely scaling) dermatitis

Some people may have a condition where large areas of the body are affected by dermatitis. It may happen that the underlying skin becomes red and overheated due to increased blood flow. Very large quantities of the skin may be shed very quickly, just like a tree shedding leaves in the autumn – which is why the process is termed exfoliative. If you should be unfortunate enough to have this type, you will require special medical and nursing supervision, because sudden changes in body temperature may occur frequently and rapidly (see chapter seven).

I shall be dealing with all these eight types of dermatitis at greater length in the course of the book, and in chapters four and five I shall describe the various tests and treatments that help to control and alleviate inflammation of the skin. Research into possible causes of dermatitis will be examined in chapter eight. But first, I want to look in detail at dermatitis in babies, children and adolescents, who together form the most commonly affected section of the population.

2 FROM BIRTH TO ADOLESCENCE

The young child with dermatitis

Dermatitis in young children is a common problem. As many as 40 per cent of children attending skin clinics in children's hospitals may have dermatitis in one form or another. In contrast, despite the fact that adults have more problems with the many materials they handle in the course of their occupations the proportion of people with dermatitis attending adult clinics is usually lower. This shows that in most cases the child will 'grow out of it' – good news for all parents, but at times difficult to believe when you're coping at three o'clock in the morning with a cross, miserable, scratching child!

Although very few children are actually born with dermatitis, a small proportion develop their first skin problems within a month of birth. In nearly all cases they begin the same way, with patches of skin becoming red, slightly swollen, possibly with tiny blister-pimples that weep when burst and become crusted.

In most cases the patches appear to be very itchy. Even though very young babies cannot co-ordinate their limbs to allow them to scratch, you can see clearly that they do know where the itch is and try to deal with it by rubbing their cheek or whatever part of the body is affected against their pillow or coverlet. By about two to three months, the ability to scratch is developed and you can see your baby's small fingers scratching at the affected areas. The most obvious times are when clothes are removed, and sometimes after a bath, when the skin is warm.

Although some children have contact dermatitis, the vast majority of sufferers are adults and so this type is covered in the next chapter. Of the three commonest types of dermatitis found in very young children, two rarely persist beyond the first year, and I shall deal with these first.

OVERLEAF: As many as one child in ten under five years old may have atopic dermatitis. Fortunately, far fewer older school children are affected.

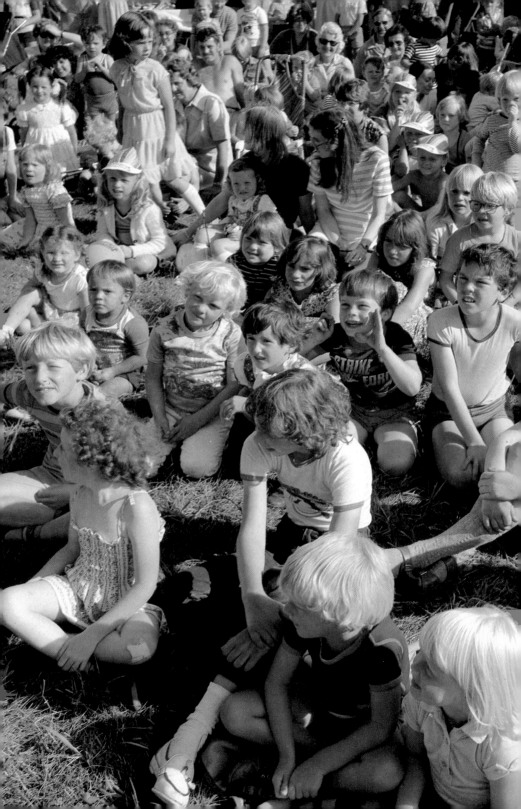

Infantile seborrhoeic dermatitis

We cannot say for certain why such small children should suddenly develop this skin condition. Often there is no history of dermatitis either in the parents or in the immediate family.

It generally appears first as a rash on baby's head and soon the scalp is covered with yellow greasy scales – known as cradle cap. Usually red scaly areas then develop on the child's body especially in the skin folds and on the face. There is no doubt that when this form of dermatitis is severe the sight of baby's skin and scalp can be very distressing to new parents. Surprisingly the child himself will appear quite content and eat and sleep normally.

We know from experience that in nearly all cases the dermatitis will have disappeared by the age of around one year and often earlier, helped of course with shampoos, creams and ointments. There are some excellent over-the-counter preparations available, but in severe cases your family doctor may prescribe a stronger remedy. We have not been able to come up with any evidence that diet plays any part in this type of dermatitis (see page 75) and a baby can, therefore, be bottle fed or introduced to mixed feeding, according to the normal

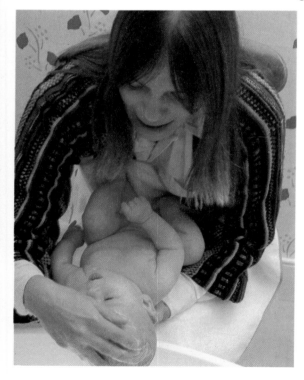

There are many excellent over-the-counter shampoos available that will help to clear cradle cap.

family pattern.

Napkin dermatitis (nappy or diaper rash)

This is a very common problem in young babies and is the result of prolonged contact between baby's sensitive skin and urine-soaked napkins. You will notice small red pimples and patches of rough skin developing on your child's buttocks and thighs. If baby has a tendency to frequent and loose bowel movements the problem can be more difficult to clear, as organisms from the bowel break down constituents of the urine to cause even more skin irritation. Some children are more likely to get this form of dermatitis than others and there is some tendency for it to run in families.

The cure is to keep the skin of the napkin area permanently clean and dry – not an easy task! You may be given protective creams and ointments to place on the affected area by your own doctor. The

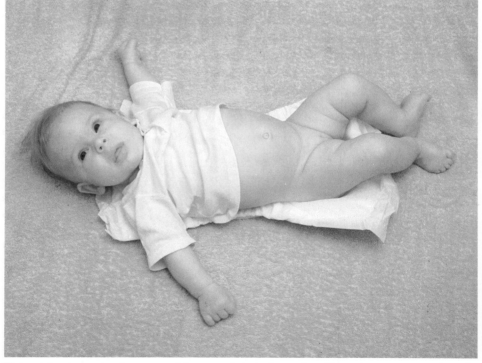

The quickest way to clear nappy/diaper rash is to keep the affected parts exposed to air for as long as possible.

quickest way to help them work is to forget about waterproof pants completely and keep baby in a warm room lying on top of a napkin – either cloth or disposable – which you should change as soon as it becomes soiled or wet. Do not wrap a napkin around the child.

Although this way of treating napkin rash is time-consuming and will mean a lot of washing for you if you don't use disposables, it is extremely effective. Exposing the rash to the air is one sure way of curing it. Once the dermatitis is healed, a normal napkin/diaper routine can be resumed, but with more frequent changes and less use of waterproof pants than before the problem developed.

It's important that cloth napkins are thoroughly rinsed after washing or soaking in antiseptic solution, since if any remains and comes in contact with baby's skin it is likely to aggravate the condition of the skin.

Atopic dermatitis (childhood eczema)

This is the commonest and best-known form of dermatitis in children, and is what most people think of when they talk of 'eczema'. In fact, 90 per cent of children with dermatitis have the atopic type, and it is estimated that it affects 3 per cent of all British babies. Comparatively very few adults have atopic dermatitis and that is why it is appropriate to concentrate on the condition in this chapter.

The first signs of the problem usually develop when the child is between two and six months old. In many families other members are also affected and parents will recognize the early signs only too well. If only one parent has a personal or family history of asthma, hay fever, or atopic dermatitis then the children are no more likely to have problems than those whose parents have no history of these diseases. If, however, both parents have one or more of these diseases in their families, then the chances of similar problems in their children are increased.

These three associated problems, atopic dermatitis, asthma and hay fever (known collectively as 'atopy') are in fact extremely common in Europe and North America and as many as 10 per cent of the population are affected. In many babies the problems are mild and the affected infants lose all trace of their dermatitis before their second birthday. In a small number, though, it is more persistent and lasts through babyhood, childhood and into adolescence in spite of treatment.

The early signs

The first signs of atopic dermatitis will be a restless, fretful baby obviously trying to rub his head or his back against the cot or crib. You will begin to discover scratch marks on and around the affected areas once he has learnt to co-ordinate his fingers. The red, weeping, crusted patches may appear on any part of the body, but in a young infant, the cheeks and the areas behind the ears are most frequently involved. Occasionally it affects the head, but unlike the greasy scaling of cradle cap, it is usually seen as a widespread crusting of head and face. For the toddler the wrists and ankles are common sites and for the older child the areas behind the knees and in the folds of the elbows are usually most affected.

Do be extra vigilant about cutting nails – a young baby's nails may grow very rapidly. Sharp fingernails at any age can turn patches of dermatitis into unpleasant infected scratch marks.

Diet and atopic dermatitis

The relationship between diet and atopic dermatitis is currently the subject of much research. As yet no clear guidelines can be given about allergies and the food we eat but if you have a family history of atopy, it is good practice to give your baby only breast milk if possible and to delay introducing supplementary milk feeds and mixed feeding. I shall be discussing allergic reaction to certain types of food at the end of this chapter, and be giving more detailed advice on diet in chapter six.

Learning to cope with it

There is no doubt that a young infant with a skin problem can cause distress and disruption to other members of the family. It may be that your first baby develops the disorder. Like many new mothers you may be very concerned that the unsightly redness and scaling on your child's skin is somehow the result of your own lack of experience. This is not the case. All types of dermatitis seen in infants are just as common in second, third or fourth children as they are in firstborn.

Atopic dermatitis may affect your baby's sleeping habits and he will tend to wake other family members throughout the night. Although exhausting and trying for parents, it is nevertheless important to create as calm an atmosphere as possible around your restless, irritable child. There is no doubt that even very young children are able to sense tension around them, and this can further aggravate the problem.

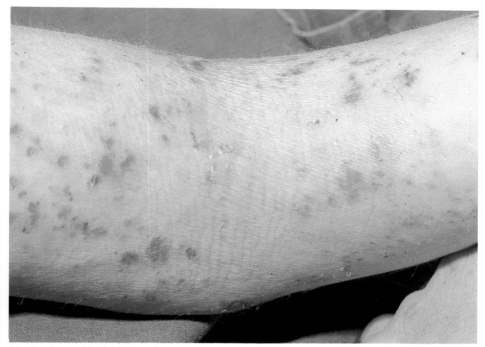
Atopic dermatitis (childhood eczema).

Seek help early

In all patients with dermatitis and particularly with small children, it is important to seek professional medical help as early on in the disease as possible. New types of cream and ointment and new approaches to treatment are regularly being introduced and you will want to take full benefit of these. One word of warning here, though. Don't apply cream or ointment prescribed for another family member to your baby's skin. This might make matters very much worse – a preparation suitable for use on the thicker skin of an adult could damage the much thinner and more sensitive skin of a young baby (see chapter five).

Keeping clean

If your baby has dermatitis, you may have to make some adjustments to the routine of the daily bath. While children with seborrhoeic dermatitis and nappy or diaper rash will enjoy and benefit from their bath, some young children with atopic dermatitis will have very dry skin and appear to be particularly uncomfortable and irritable after their bath. If you find this happening cut bath time to once or twice weekly and keep your child clean between bathing with a simple sponging down.

Soap and even some of the special infant bath 'additives' can irritate dry sensitive skin, so you may be advised to use only moisturizing oils which your family doctor will recommend for you. Many young children with atopic dermatitis feel much better if you abandon soap altogether and instead clean their skin with an emulsifying ointment. If soap is necessary don't use a highly scented variety, as it may irritate the skin.

If you observe these simple methods of minimizing the chances of your baby being exposed to irritant materials, and a cleansing routine is developed which in effect replaces and supplements the film of natural oils on the child's skin, then many young children with atopic dermatitis will be relatively comfortable and outgrow their condition before they reach school age. An unfortunate few will, however, continue to have problems and the care of this group will be considered next.

The school child with dermatitis

Those school-aged children who have dermatitis are more likely to have the atopic type of dermatitis than any of the other kinds and you will usually find that they have had skin problems since early infancy. In fact, a recent study found that one out of every hundred British school children has atopic dermatitis.

Five-year-olds tend to have dry, scaly atopic dermatitis with some thickening of the skin in the elbow creases and behind the knees. Itch is a problem and this may make concentration difficult in the classroom. If the itch keeps your child awake at night he will probably be tired and listless in class, and if he is receiving an anti-itch antihistamine syrup to help control the itch at night, he may be difficult to waken for school in the morning.

Although very few five-year-olds are self-conscious about their 'different' skin they may rapidly become so if there are any thoughtless remarks or teasing from other children. It would be wise in any case to prepare your child for some of the remarks he is likely to get from other children who have never seen skin problems.

Preparation builds confidence
Tell your child that his skin problem is a nuisance but that with care and treatment it will improve and one day clear up completely. He

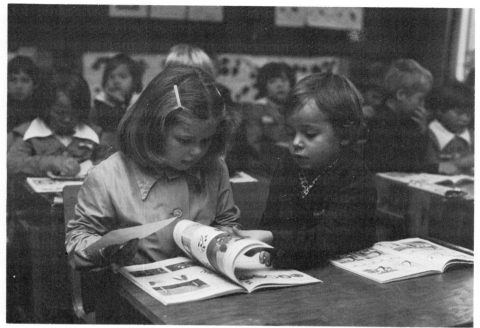

If your school child has atopic dermatitis, make sure the teachers know that she shouldn't sit by a sunny window or radiator.

will not pass it on to his friends, and as long as his skin is not chapped or sore, he can do almost all the things the other children do. If his hands are very dry and chapped then tell him not to play with sand or water, and if you have noticed signs of reactions to animal hair, he should be told not to go near any furry pets kept in the classroom.

A brief chat with your child's teacher will also help prevent any misunderstanding. Explain that this is not an infectious or contagious problem. Explain also that children with dermatitis should not become overheated as this makes their skin very uncomfortable. It helps if they can have a chair well away from the radiator or a sunny window. But apart from these precautions the child should take part in all the activities of the class, including sports.

Learning to swim is an important activity for all young children whether organized by the school or by parents. The child with dermatitis should not be excluded. Careful showering after using the swimming baths will prevent the chlorine that is used in the water as a disinfectant from irritating the skin. At the seaside your child

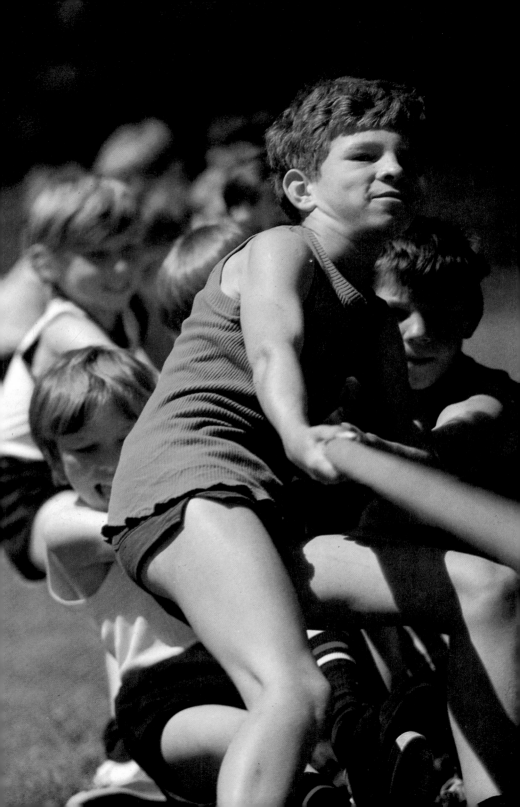

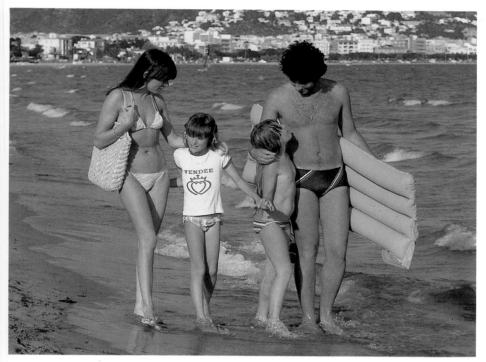

ABOVE: Many children's atopic dermatitis improves when on a sunny seaside vacation.
OPPOSITE: There's no reason why children with atopic dermatitis shouldn't participate in sports. It will do wonders for their morale.

may find that the salt sea water may sting the areas of dermatitis at first, but many children actually experience clearing of their dermatitis during a holiday at the seaside. It is not known whether this is due to the sea water, fresh air, the additional sunshine, the general feeling of family relaxation, or a happy mixture of all these ingredients.

It is difficult to give useful guidelines as to when a school child is likely to outgrow dermatitis, but many do so at the age of puberty – around twelve to fourteen years. In fact, 80 per cent of young children grow out of atopic dermatitis. This should give both you and your school child encouragement and hope.

The adolescent and dermatitis

There are always the unfortunate few who continue to have derma-

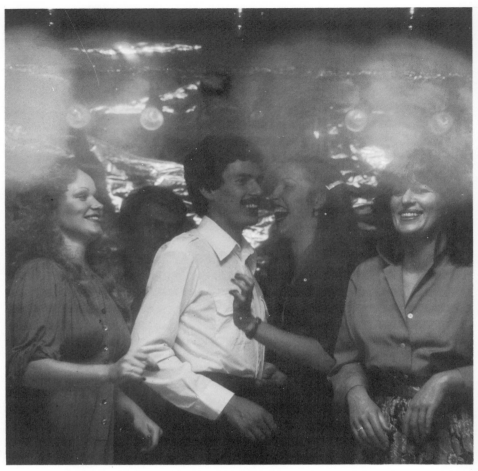

Teenagers with atopic dermatitis should be encouraged to socialize. Jeans and long-sleeved shirts will usually hide the problem.

titis, and even some who develop dermatitis at adolescence, and they deserve special consideration and attention. Adolescence can be a stormy and difficult time for many teenagers and a time when the desire to form part of a group or a crowd is very strong. There's nothing like sore, red, itchy skin and the paraphernalia of messy preparations and bandages to make a teenager feel different and an outcast – feelings which are usually much more strongly experienced by the sufferer than by his friends. Because of this, it is all too easy for teenagers with atopic dermatitis to become withdrawn and depressed.

The important thing is for parents to be aware of this and to encourage a cheerful, hopeful approach that things will improve. Although self-consciousness may make the teenager very reluctant to take part in normal social gatherings, he or she should be encouraged to do so. Attractive long-sleeved shirts or blouses and the normal teenage uniform of blue jeans will hide most of the problem. Remind your child that famous athletes like Alan Pascoe and Dawn Fraser have had the related problem of asthma – and overcome it. Always push home the message: Keep treating your skin and keep cheerful! It is certainly worth encouraging your child to continue treatment, as eventually the dermatitis will improve.

Does stress cause dermatitis?

While tension and stress won't actually cause dermatitis, they can certainly aggravate it. Defining stress is difficult, as we all worry about different things. One person can cope apparently easily with circumstances that for another would be an intolerable burden.

One of the most likely causes of stress in school children and students is, of course, examinations. Anyone with atopic dermatitis should be encouraged to try to approach all examinations as calmly as possible; undue parental pressure to succeed is rarely an effective stimulus, and if your child has dermatitis, it could well make matters worse. As your child begins preparing for exams it will be of value to explain to teachers that the child is regularly attending his family doctor or a skin specialist. It is particularly important to tell the teaching staff if your child is receiving antihistamine or other pills as they may cause slight drowsiness in class, which could be confused with lack of interest or attention.

When a stay in hospital is necessary

Although it is general policy on the part of most dermatologists to treat young children as out-patients whenever possible, older children with chronic dermatitis in a particularly acute and uncomfortable phase will often benefit from a short period of care in a hospital ward. The improvement seen after such an admission may not always be long-lived, but it will certainly improve morale and convince your child that with regular treatment his skin can look normal.

Two particular points which may be of value during such a hospital admission are first, practical demonstration by skilled nurses of exactly how to apply the creams and ointments prescribed; and second, a chance to compare his own skin problems with those of sufferers from other conditions such as psoriasis. The realization that skin disease is not a great rarity will make it easier for the child to cope with his own condition. You may find national patients' associations to be of great psychological support as well as offering practical and helpful advice. A list of useful addresses has been included at the end of the book.

Other problems that may be associated with atopic dermatitis

Atopic dermatitis may be associated with a variety of other problems, some related to the skin and others to quite different parts of the body. I shall deal first with those that most people will immediately link with atopic dermatitis, or childhood eczema, as it is also called.

Atopy: the threefold affliction

Three different conditions make up the group of diseases called atopy. These are asthma, hay fever (allergic rhinitis), and dermatitis. Many people only suffer from one of these conditions, but others have two or even a 'full house', with all three present. Unfair as it may seem, not only does atopic dermatitis have a tendency to run in families, but usually a family with one of the diseases will have the other two as well! A parent, for instance, may have severe hay fever, one child asthma and another dermatitis.

According to a recent study in the United States, up to 20 per cent of the population has a combination of atopic dermatitis, asthma and hay fever. At present there is no way of telling in early infancy who will develop hay fever, who will develop dermatitis and who asthma. In general, dermatitis is the commonest form of atopy in young children, and hay fever is commoner in adults.

Asthma
Allergic asthma can start at any age, but around 30 per cent of cases are among children under ten years old. It is a particularly annoying problem for those children of school age who are keen to join in all the usual sporting activities. With proper care and management this can often be done – some well-known Olympic athletes and other sportsmen are asthmatics and knowledge of this can be very encouraging to the young sufferer.

Asthma is easily recognized as a tightness of the chest and a difficulty in breathing deeply. In normal breathing, the phase of breathing out lasts longer than breathing in but in people with asthma it's the other way around. A feeling of not being able to breathe, of tightness or of choking, is naturally an alarming one for anyone, particularly a child. It is also extremely distressing for parents to have to watch their child having a wheezing attack. The symptoms are often made very much worse by the common cold which in asthmatics tends to become centred in the chest.

In the past ten years methods of treating asthmatic attacks and, more important, of preventing them from happening, have become very much better with the new and very effective preventive drugs now available. Dr Allan Knight's *Asthma and Hay Fever*, in this Positive Health Guide series, is particularly useful for people with either of these ailments.

Hay fever (allergic rhinitis) Young adults are the group who seem to suffer most from hay fever, and some of them may have had atopic dermatitis in infancy. The symptoms of hay fever are caused by an allergy or hypersensitivity to pollens in the air, which are usually at their worst in the spring and early summer. You will develop severe and irritating bouts of sneezing accompanied by streaming eyes and nose and the general appearance of a severe head cold.

The condition varies in severity from one season to the next, with the worst episodes usually associated with high pollen counts. These are a measure of the number of pollen grains in the air, and may be recorded in the daily newspapers or reported on radio or television. Different types of grasses may be responsible, such as rye or timothy grasses, and symptoms may appear or disappear very rapidly if you move to an area in which the type of grass causing this particular problem is more or less common.

It is possible to identify the grass or grasses that cause your hay fever by blood tests, and in some cases a desensitizing mixture can be prepared. This will be given to you as a series of injections (usually six given at weekly intervals) in the winter months. In many cases the results have been good with an absence of symptoms, or at least an improvement, over the following spring and summer. The injections normally have to be repeated each year and the dosage increased. Unfortunately, no such desensitizing procedure has been shown to be useful for atopic dermititis.

Dry skin (xerosis) and 'fish' skin (ichthyosis)
A large number of people with atopic dermatitis have a tendency to dry skin which is flaky and tends to crack and chap in cold weather. Many of them also have rough areas like permanent 'goose pimples' on the outer part of their upper arms. The medical term for this is

keratosis pilaris, and it is really more of a nuisance or of cosmetic importance – certainly not a severe problem. You can control the roughness by rubbing the affected parts of your body with a loofah and then applying a lubricating cream.

About half of all people who suffer from atopic dermatitis have this dry skin and in some the fine scaling is so severe that doctors call the condition 'ichthyosis'. This term means, literally, 'fish skin' and is a good description of the very obvious scaliness which may be present.

This kind of extreme dryness tends to be more of a problem in early childhood and usually improves around puberty. Your teenage children with atopic dermatitis and dry skin can take some comfort from the fact that they are unlikely to suffer from a common problem of their age group – acne, which is seen more often in those with greasy skin.

Fungal infections
Many people have had fungal infections at some time, but there is evidence that people with atopic dermatitis are even more likely to have this form of infection. Athlete's foot (tinea pedis), is a particularly common type of fungus infection. Simple preventive measures are to make sure you dry the skin between the toes carefully and thoroughly, and use one of the antifungal dusting powders available at chemists and pharmacies.

'Allergy' to food
Increasingly in recent years doctors are being asked whether there is a relationship between diet and atopic dermatitis. Undoubtedly a considerable number of people with this form of dermatitis find they cannot take certain foods. Eggs, for example, will make them sick, or fish will cause swelling and tingling of the lips and the inside of their mouth. They have an 'allergy', they say, to these particular foods. But the word 'allergy' means a very specific type of reaction and as not all these food-related reactions are true allergies, the term 'food intolerance' is more accurate than 'food allergy' for this condition. As it turns out, most of the foods that cause these reactions are protein foods and it is usually a very particular kind of protein – for example, it may be related to egg white but not to egg yolk, or to egg yolk in the raw state but not in the cooked state. In young children these food intolerance problems are often temporary, so if your child is regularly sick when given egg yolk, don't assume that he will not be able to eat eggs for the rest of his life. Try reintroducing

the food in small quantities after an interval of three to six months.

In chapter six I shall be giving further advice on diet for young dermatitis sufferers, as well as a variety of practical suggestions for making life easier for them, including ideas for clothing, careers and ways to arrange the home. But now I want to move on to look at how dermatitis can affect adults.

3 ADULTS AND DERMATITIS

Dermatitis can affect any of us at varying stages in our lives. One of the features of modern life is the enormous variety of materials we have to come into contact with, not only in our places of work but in our homes, too. Hardly surprisingly many of these materials – some natural, some synthetic – either damage or irritate our skin and trigger off a reaction within our bodies. The result is contact dermatitis, which is the type that affects eight out of every ten adults with dermatitis. There are other types of dermatitis in adults, including seborrhoeic dermatitis, which may be associated with severe dandruff, and varicose dermatitis of the older person. Adults can also have atopic dermatitis, but this is mostly a younger person's problem and so has been covered in the previous chapter.

Irritant contact dermatitis caused by frequent immersion in soapy water – known as 'washerwoman's hands'.

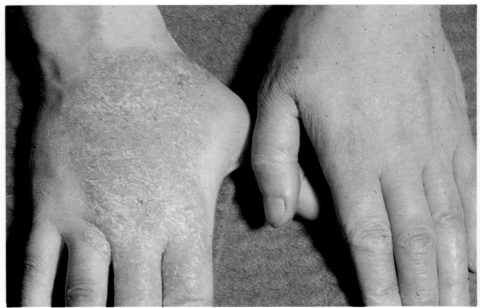

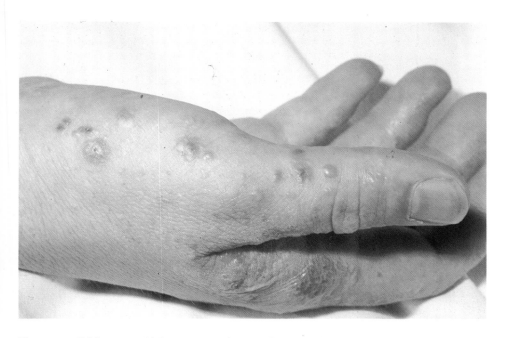

These small blisters, which are sometimes a feature of irritant contact dermatitis, are called pompholyx.

But whatever the cause of the dermatitis, remember that in almost every case our skin reacts in much the same way as I described in chapter one and goes through the three stages of acute, subacute and chronic if the cause is not discovered and removed and no treatment is given.

Irritant contact dermatitis

This is the commonest type of dermatitis in adult life. It may trouble some 5 per cent of the population, according to a recent Swedish study, with even higher percentages in certain trades: 8 per cent of building workers and 12 per cent of furniture workers, for example.

This variety of contact dermatitis is due to irritant materials that cause the skin to become inflamed. Tiny blisters that look like sago grains (and are known as pompholyx) may then develop. This is particularly noticeable where the film of thin but very valuable fatty material (lipid) on the surface of normal healthy skin has been destroyed by detergents and other degreasing agents. Once this important protective barrier has gone and your skin is left dry and chapped from constant immersion in water and detergents, irritant dermatitis has a higher chance of developing. The typical wear-and-tear dermatitis caused by this is most frequently seen on the hands and is known as 'washerwoman's hands', although it is not confined to women and can be caused by other materials than soap, detergent and water: by anything, in fact, that removes or attacks the skin's fatty film. Irritant contact dermatitis is particulary likely to affect you if you spend time working in cold windy conditions with wet skin.

Who is likely to develop irritant contact dermatitis?
Housewives with young children are very much at risk from this kind of dermatitis due to working with their hands in water. Cleaners and domestic workers are also at risk as they are in constant contact with detergents and other degreasing materials. Hospital work is also a high-risk occupation. Another is hairdressing, where much of your time as a junior is spent shampooing and working with permanent-wave lotions. Wearing rubber gloves can help in all these occupa-

Hairdressers are particularly prone to irritant contact dermatitis.

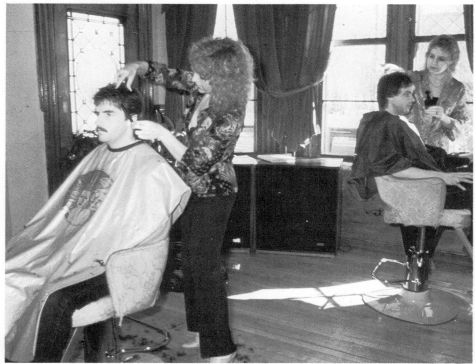

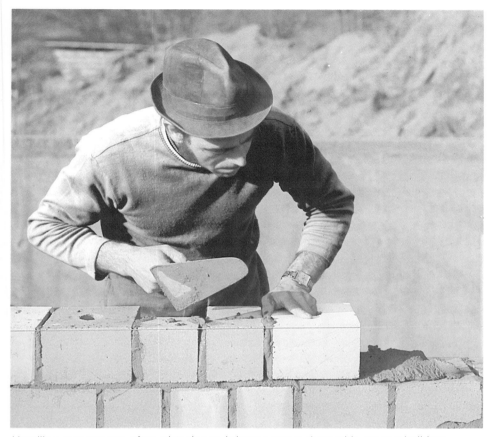
Handling cement can often give rise to irritant contact dermatitis among builders.

tions, although these too can cause irritation. Using proprietary moisturizing lotions and protective barrier creams is a good way of keeping damage to the hands to a minimum (see page 65).

Workers in the textile and rubber industries may be in contact with many irritants and even such apparently 'safe' occupations as floristry are not without risk as some common fertilizers may irritate the skin. In Scandinavia, caterers who arrange the ingredients on the open sandwiches with such artistry often develop problems with hand dermatitis as a result of handling a variety of pickled food, as well as constant hand-washing.

Other occupations and hobbies that carry a high risk of irritant contact dermatitis include the building industry (from cement), handling and manufacturing plastics and rubber, car repair work, interior decorating, woodwork, marquetry and car maintenance.

Allergic, or sensitization, contact dermatitis

This is the name given to the second variety of contact dermatitis, which is caused by a group of white blood cells, the T lymphocytes, becoming sensitized to an 'allergen' – a material that can cause an allergy. It affects more women than men; one Swedish study showed that 10 per cent of women had allergic dermatitis, and only 2 per cent of men.

First signs of acute allergic contact dermatitis are itching, redness, tiny blisters and moist patches. Small blisters may develop on hands and feet; this picture may also occur in various other types of dermatitis and may be intensely itchy. As the condition becomes more chronic, dryness and scaliness will develop and may become permanent.

There are a very large number of materials that can act as allergens and trigger off allergic contact dermatitis. As if that were not enough, a further group of materials, such as the metal nickel, while not

Allergic contact dermatitis caused by detergent in a bra strap.

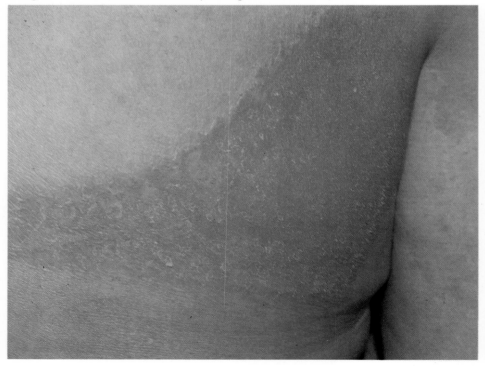

actually allergens themselves, become so when linked to protein material in our skin.

In allergic contact dermatitis, a rash may take a week or more to appear after the first contact with whatever is acting as the allergen. On the other hand, you may handle a material – rubber, nickel, cement, say – for many years with no problems and then suddenly break out in a rash. As you can imagine, this makes tracking down the cause doubly difficult as probably you, and indeed your doctor, will be much more inclined to blame materials that are new to your environment.

To confuse matters further, once allergic contact dermatitis has developed, it can affect any part of your skin and not just where you made contact with the sensitizing material, and the rash that develops may be very widespread. Normally, though, whatever parts of your body touched the substance are the first to be affected and usually more severely than anywhere else. These points are important in tracking down the material responsible. The reaction can be triggered off again in special tests using exactly the same substance that caused the dermatitis in the first place – although occasionally two closely related substances may show cross-reactivity. There is a good example of this among some people – mostly women – who have allergic dermatitis due to the metal nickel. In many cases testing shows that these people are also sensitive to chromium.

Once you have contracted this type of allergy, you usually remain sensitive to the particular material for life. Unfortunately, also, only very small amounts of the material are needed to set off the rash again after the first episode. I remember treating a man for dermatitis of the upper leg and as we talked I discovered that he was a policeman and the dermatitis was due to the nickel in the handcuffs in his pocket. So even indirect contact between handcuffs – or, more commonly, metal coins – in a trouser pocket and the underlying skin may be enough to provoke a generalized rash.

What are the danger materials?
Most substances that cause allergic contact dermatitis can be handled perfectly safely by the majority of people. Some of the better-known potential causes of this dermatitis, such as rubber, nickel and hair dyes, are quite safe for most people, but a smaller group of materials act as allergens on a large number of people. An example of this group are the epoxy-resin chemicals which are found in many modern adhesives. Fairly large numbers of people develop reactions to these, especially when the manufacturer's instructions about safety

are not followed. (See the table on pages 46 and 47.)

For women, the commonest type of allergic contact dermatitis arises as a result of sensitivity to nickel. Nickel, of course, is an extremely common material, and is found on so many things: clothing (nickel clips and hooks), on jewellery (earrings), in the kitchen (cutlery, sinks, and pots and pans), in the office (door knobs, typewriter keys), in the car, in coins and mixed in with many other materials. In short, it is virtually impossible *not* to come into contact with nickel at some time in your life.

Other commonly found sensitizers are hair dye; rubber and elastic materials, used in underclothes and rubber gloves; chromates used in tanning leather, for belts, shoes and bags; adhesive resins, widely used in the home and in the manufacture of shoes; and some plants, particularly the indoor pot plant primula obconica.

For men, the commonest sensitizers are found in the cement widely used in the building industry, as well as epoxy resin adhesives, rubber chemicals, and many of the materials mentioned above. Sensitivity to nickel, though, is largely a women's problem.

Who is likely to develop allergic contact dermatitis?
The answer to this question is rather complicated. Obviously, just as various materials differ in the degree of sensitization they are able to inflict, so we as unique individuals differ in our susceptibility to sensitization. Also, an important feature of allergic contact dermatitis is that the material responsible for the trouble is quite harmless to most people. A number of substances which don't cause sensitization in 95 per cent of the population will cause allergic contact dermatitis in the remaining 5 per cent, should they touch them.

A great many of those who develop allergic contact dermatitis do so in the course of their hobbies or even as a result of clothing worn regularly. This is worth remembering, for this type of dermatitis is often associated with work, but substances at home can be just as important.

How do you know if you have allergic contact dermatitis?
1. The most important point here is to think back very carefully to when the dermatitis first developed and in what part of your body. This will be a most important clue, and time spent remembering these details is not wasted.
2. If the rash temporarily improves while you're away from home

then you can suspect some material or materials within your home. 3. If it improves when you are away from your regular employment (it may be a week before any noticeable improvement), then material handled at work may be responsible.

What action should you take?

After some detective work of this kind to identify the likely culprit, the next step is to keep away from the suspected object or material causing the problem so that your skin can settle down and return to normal. You will, I hope, be in contact with your doctor and the creams and ointments he gives you will speed up the return to normal. Of course, if you can't avoid contact with the material, the 'settling down' period may be prolonged indefinitely.

When your skin is relatively normal, your dermatologist may apply what are known as 'patch tests' – small patches containing tiny quantities of the suspect material in different concentrations – to your skin, usually on your back (see chapter four).

The tests will be carried out by a skin specialist, often at a special contact dermatitis clinic. It may be necessary for you to attend the clinic several times so that you can give the doctor a good history of the development of the condition, before he carries out the tests. Doctors and nurses in these clinics are very skilled at the detective work needed to track down the cause of contact dermatitis and will often pin-point a possible source of trouble that you had not thought important.

This routine of patch testing sounds very simple, but there are many pitfalls and it is most unwise to try to carry out a makeshift patch test at home. The materials you use may be in too strong a concentration which, put on sore and inflamed skin, will result in a very severe reaction. This test is best left to the experts who know exactly how and when to carry it out.

What to do at work

A common and important problem is what kind of action to take when patch tests show that you have developed a contact dermatitis due to sensitization to material handled in the course of your work. Your employer, factory doctor or industrial medical officer can all be of great help in this situation and it may be quite possible for you to switch to a different type of work in the same office or factory without having to leave your firm. Certainly at a time of growing unemployment this solution is much the most satisfactory for any employee. Check, though, that it is the occupation itself, and not

Common materials responsible for allergic contact dermatitis

Rubber and rubber-associated chemicals	Rubber gloves, rubber boots, parts on normal shoes, insoles, imitation leather watch straps.
Nickel	Very many materials including stainless steel; kitchen tools; pots; pans; cutlery; jewellery (even gold and silver may contain a proportion of nickel as a hardener); fastenings on clothing, zips, metal watches and straps; coins; door knobs; arch supports in shoes; car handles; gear levers. Nickel can even be absorbed in very small amounts from food.
Chromium and chromates	All leather (chromium is used in tanning), gloves, watch straps, shoes, paints, printing work, cement (particularly wet mortar), some metal hooks.
Synthetic plastics and resins (Epoxy resins)	Glues, 'hardeners', insulating materials. All footwear contains layers of materials glued together; many of these glues may cause problems.
Lanolin, and preservatives used in cosmetics and prescribed creams	Cosmetics, proprietary creams and ointments. Especially: parabens – a preservative; Neomycin – an antibiotic; and antihistamine – an anti-itch preparation. Antihistamines should be taken by mouth, not applied to the skin. Antibiotics other than Neomycin are less likely to cause allergy.
Hair dyes	Those containing para phenylene diamine (PPD). Check the packet.
Plants	Primula obconica (*opposite left*), cineraria and chrysanthemum (*opposite right*); poison ivy (rhus toxicodendron) and poison sumach (rhus vernix) – mainly North America; and Japanese wax tree (rhus succedanum) and grevillea – mainly Australia.

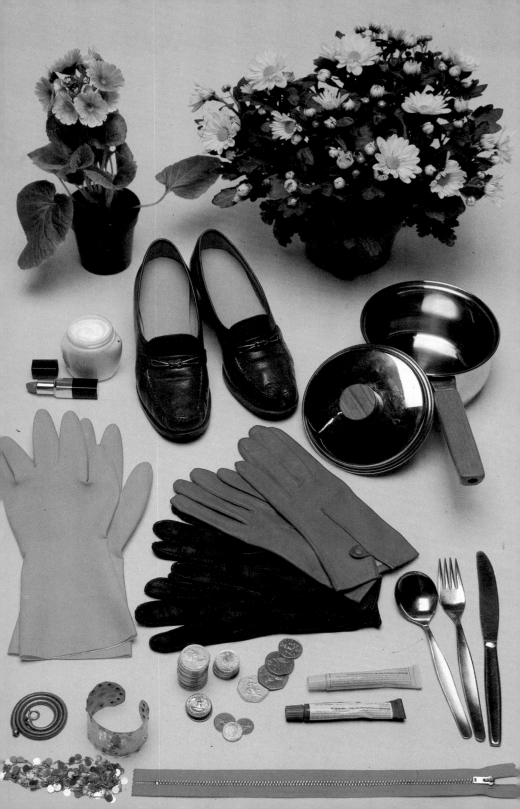

some related material that is the problem, as the following case illustrates:

Sarah Baxter, a young woman who worked in the textile industry, came to our clinic with severe dermatitis of her hands which, she said, was worse when she was at work and improved greatly when she was away from work either ill or on holiday. While at work she handled large quantities of cloth daily. Naturally, it was assumed that her dermatitis was due to the cloth she handled but patch tests showed that she was sensitive to nickel. Then we discovered that because she worked in a very hot, dry, dusty environment, she kept a mug of water beside her and drank from it regularly. The mug was made partly of the culprit material nickel. When she changed over to a plastic mug her hands healed up considerably and she was able to continue in her old job.

It would be equally wrong to assume that if several people working together have dermatitis, their problems are all due to the same cause or the same material at work. It is quite possible for one of them to have hand problems due to nickel, another to have a dermatitis due to epoxy resin glues used in do-it-yourself activities at weekends and yet another to have dermatitis due to the colour developer he uses for his photography practised as a hobby or extra weekend job.

To sum up then, here are a few do's and don'ts for those who have allergic contact dermatitis. (For further practical suggestions see chapter six.)

Do
1. See your family doctor and co-operate with any tests he or she may ask you to undergo.
2. Tell him when you first developed the dermatitis and where on your body it first appeared.
3. Try avoiding the materials you suspect are causing your dermatitis, and note whether this has any beneficial effect (this can take up to a week). Refer to the list of common allergens on the previous spread.
4. Think carefully about new substances that you have handled recently – either at work or in the course of hobbies or recreational activities.
5. Continue to follow your doctor's prescribed treatment for your skin until the dermatitis is cleared up.

Don't

1. Jump to hasty conclusions about what may be causing your dermatitis.
2. Try to carry out patch tests on yourself.
3. Use creams or ointments that haven't been prescribed for your dermatitis. Some can actually be allergens themselves.

Adult seborrhoeic dermatitis

This is usually a mild though often chronic and rather stubborn type of dermatitis, most active on parts of our bodies with large numbers of grease-producing sebaceous glands – the scalp, face, upper part of the chest and between the shoulder blades. People who are affected by this disease are usually male and between twenty and thirty years old.

There is actually no direct evidence to link sebaceous glands with adult seborrhoeic dermatitis. Nor is there any evidence to link the

Adult seborrhoeic dermatitis often affects the scalp.

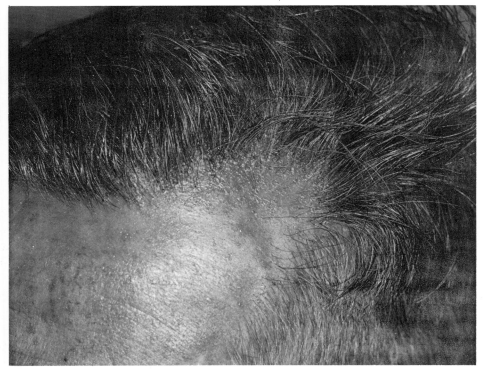

adult condition with infant seborrhoeic dermatitis, or cradle cap, which we discussed in chapter two. The cause of adult seborrhoeic dermatitis is not yet understood, though various theories linking the condition with diet, sun exposure and minor infection have been suggested. It was a condition specialists had to treat fairly frequently thirty to forty years ago, then it became quite rare and now seems to be becoming more common again.

Who gets it?
The people who are affected are usually fair haired and fair skinned. They tend to have persistent fine scaling of their scalp causing dandruff, and the underlying scalp may be red and itchy. Other areas most commonly involved are around the ears, the face, the front of the chest and under the arms. Usually all that is seen is a mild redness, and the discomfort felt by the sufferer may seem to be out of proportion to the visible rash.

Although it looks a mild and easily treatable form of dermatitis, it is, in fact, difficult to clear completely. Be careful with the preparations your doctor prescribes, as it is very easy to treat it too enthusiastically, and this will only cause further redness and irritation. It is easy, too, for the skin to become infected if you have a severe case of seborrhoeic dermatitis; and this may give rise to considerable problems with shaving if that part of your face is involved. It's worth experimenting with shaving methods as people's skin differs; you might even try growing a beard. Scaling, irritation and crusting around the eyebrows and eyelashes with sore, sticky eyes, especially first thing in the morning, are also sometimes one of the hazards of this form of dermatitis. If this is a problem, try bathing your eyes in cold water.

Varicose (stasis) dermatitis

Whereas atopic dermatitis is commonest among children and contact dermatitis is most frequently seen during adult working life, varicose dermatitis tends to be a problem for the older person. The seeds of the problem, however, have often been sown in early adult life.

One of the penalties we pay for being the most highly developed mammal and walking upright, rather than on all fours, is that the blood supply pumped around by the heart is relatively slow and sluggish in returning from the legs back to the heart for recirculation. This, of course, is because the force of gravity is acting against the pumping action of our circulatory system pushing the blood back up to the heart through the veins. In healthy, active children and young adults there are no obvious problems as a result of this, but in older people, particularly those who stand still a lot, this sluggishness becomes very much worse so that in the veins on the outside of the legs, the blood may hardly move at all (stasis means stoppage). The result is varicose veins. There are other factors involved in varicose veins, of course. They are more likely to develop:

1. If your close relatives have varicose veins.
2. If you are a woman.
3. If you are overweight.
4. If you are pregnant.
5. After inflammation of the leg veins (phlebitis), which may occur independently or be associated with pregnancy.

Early surgical or injection treatment of varicose veins may result in a complete cure so they give you no further trouble. The veins that are the cause of the problems lie near the surface of the skin and are not essential for returning the venous blood of the legs to the heart. This is done mainly by the veins set more deeply within

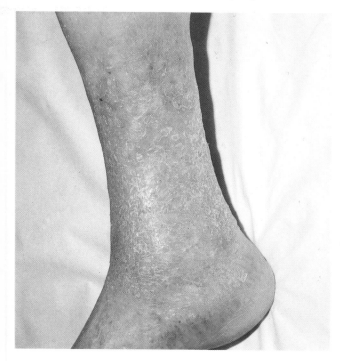

Varicose dermatitis.

51

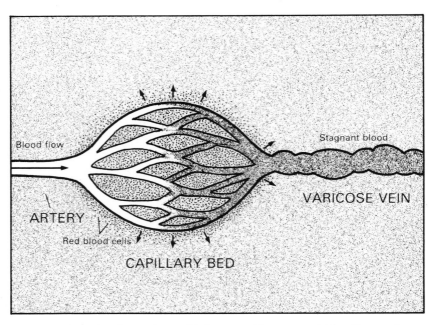

The dark colouration of varicose dermatitis is caused by stagnant blood in a varicose vein forcing red blood cells out through the thin capillaries into the surrounding skin.

your legs. It is when you ignore your varicose veins, perhaps because you're too busy to seek medical help, that the trouble continues and becomes chronic. The next stage often involves damage to the valves of the veins that connect the surface and deep veins. Surgery is then less likely to be successful.

How does varicose dermatitis develop?

When you have varicose veins, the blood flow up the leg is slow and sluggish. Fluid leaks out of blood vessels into the skin and your ankles are likely to swell, particularly in hot weather. The pressure of the blood on the walls of the veins can be very great, especially round the inside of your ankle. The skin there is likely to be starved of nourishment, becoming thin and delicate. As blood leaks through the tiny vessels, called capillaries, that link the arteries to the veins, red speckled spots will appear on the skin surface and you'll find the whole area may become inflamed and itchy.

Scratching or minor accidents, such as a knock against furniture or while getting on to a bus, may easily cause this thin unhealthy skin to break down. If this happens it is essential that you get early treatment because if you don't this may not heal and could develop into a varicose ulcer. Healing of these is a long, wearying business, with the skin constantly tending to break down again.

The first essential in this type of dermatitis is prevention. This must begin early if you have a strong family history of varicose veins. Don't let yourself get overweight and always wear elastic support stockings (which are better than tights) during either pregnancy or at work if your job involves a lot of standing.

It may be that, despite these measures, varicose veins develop. They are easily recognized by the presence of the knotted twisted blue-black veins, a feeling of 'heavy legs' and tell-tale itchy areas around your ankles. Seepage of blood from capillaries may cause the skin to become a speckled-brown colour. If you have varicose veins ask to see a surgeon as soon as possible. He (or she) will decide whether injections or surgery is the best form of treatment.

If you bump and actually damage a swollen varicose vein, you might be alarmed by the dramatic bleeding. This, though, is easily controlled. Just lie flat, raise your ankle above the level of your chest and press on the wound with a clean handkerchief or cloth. The power of gravity will quickly help prevent any further loss of blood.

Do's and don'ts

I shall discuss treatment more fully in the next chapter. Meanwhile here are a few useful points:

1. **Do** use a bandage or pad under support stockings or tights for extra protection.
2. **Don't** use creams and ointments other than those specially prescribed. Many people with varicose dermatitis develop allergic contact dermatitis as a result of applying large numbers of different preparations to the ankle area. Often it is a cause of varicose dermatitis failing to heal or becoming worse during treatment.
3. **Do** use paste bandages impregnated with soothing preparations containing tar or ichthyol. These bandages are extremely useful because they perform the double task of assisting healing and also protecting against further damage from bumps and knocks.
4. **Do** tell your doctor if any cream causes stinging or itching, or inflammation of the surrounding skin, as this may be an early sign of trouble.
5. **Do** agree to patch tests if suggested by your doctor or specialist, as these can be used to check whether or not you have developed any allergies to the many creams and ointments that have been prescribed.

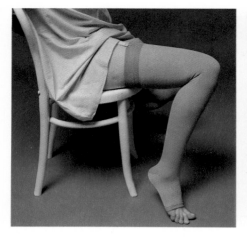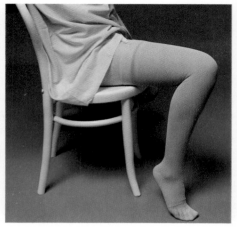

A long support stocking . . . covered by an ordinary stocking to improve appearance.

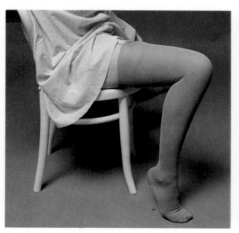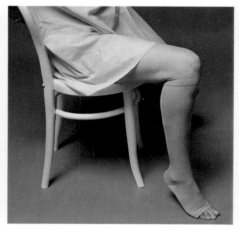

A cosmetic support stocking.   A short support stocking.

Prevention of varicose dermatitis is much better than cure. If you have varicose veins, wearing good support stockings prescribed by your doctor will help keep them under control.

Because there are so many different types of dermatitis, and indeed of other similar complaints, tests are of crucial importance in determining exactly which condition you are affected by and which treatment is right for you. The next chapter explains what these various tests involve.

4 TESTS AND INVESTIGATIONS

Although a doctor can learn a lot about a skin disease by a simple and careful inspection of your skin, it is often necessary to perform additional tests to be absolutely certain of the type of dermatitis you have – or even to distinguish between dermatitis and other common skin problems such as psoriasis.

Your family doctor or specialist will advise you if they think that a skin test is necessary, and I strongly recommend that you take their advice. No doctor undertakes unnecessary tests, particularly on small children, and although parents may find the prospect of a blood test or the removal of a small piece of their child's skin rather distressing, the child himself usually forgets the experience rapidly.

In contrast, it's quite possible that you may feel that you or your child have not received enough in the way of special tests. Your doctor will explain why they are not necessary in your case. At the present time there are no tests for telling us when a young child will grow out of atopic dermatitis. We do know that this will happen in over 80 per cent of cases but no test can tell us if this will happen when the child is two, five or ten years of age.

The range of tests which may be needed

Blood tests

These tests involve the removal of a small blood sample from one of your veins, usually in the elbow area. It may be needed for a variety of reasons, one of which is the examination of the numbers and types of white blood cells. Someone with atopic dermatitis, for instance, will often have increased numbers of a group of white blood cells, the eosinophils. Another reason for a blood test is to measure the amount of a material called immunoglobulin E (IgE) in the blood, which may be raised in atopic dermatitis. A more specialized test can detect the existence of various types of IgE that we know are directed specifically against particular allergens, such as cat hair, pollens or certain foods. This is called the RAST test. Unfortunately, even when we've identified the type of IgE and thus the materials to which you are likely to be allergic, and you manage to keep clear of them, your skin doesn't always improve. I shall be considering the importance of IgE as a possible cause of dermatitis in more detail in chapter eight. Your doctor will decide how frequently these blood tests need to be carried out, if at all.

Tests for the skin

Skin biopsy   Your specialist may want to remove a small piece of skin to be absolutely sure he knows which type of dermatitis you have. It is a very simple procedure requiring only a local anaesthetic. Two or three stitches may be needed and the whole operation takes ten to fifteen minutes.

Most dermatologists have had skin biopsies carried out on themselves and can confidently reassure you that it is not a particularly unpleasant experience – in fact, less painful than having a tooth filled at the dentist. So if your specialist advises a skin biopsy, do take his advice. You will want your specialist to have all the information he needs to make a definite diagnosis. Without a biopsy, treatment might be based partially on guesswork – never a good idea. In most cases of dermatitis, however, the diagnosis is obvious and can be made without a biopsy.

Prick tests   Long before it was possible to measure the levels of immunoglobulin E in the blood, specialists in allergic diseases used what are called 'prick tests' to give them some clues as to which substances were responsible for these allergies.

The tests involve putting one drop of a solution containing an extract of, for example, feathers, or pollen, or cat hair or one of many other substances, on the skin and then gently pricking the underlying skin with a sterile needle. If the solution contains a substance to which the patient is allergic a small raised red lump like an insect bite develops on the site of the test within ten to twenty minutes.

These tests are used more by doctors interested in respiratory allergies (such as asthma) than dermatologists but they are a rapid and easy method of obtaining information similar to that available from a blood test. Using this method it is possible to carry out tests against a very large number of substances on one visit to the clinic.

Patch tests   For anyone with suspected allergic contact dermatitis, patch tests are a common and very important part of the specialist's investigations. Although I have already mentioned them in chapter three, I will describe in detail exactly what is done as it is important to co-operate fully with your doctor over these tests.

After taking a careful history of your skin problem and examining your skin, your specialist will decide which materials are most likely to be causing the rash. The next step will be to apply an appropriate dilution of the suspected substance on a little square of lint to normal unaffected skin, usually on your back. This little patch is held in place with adhesive tape. After forty-eight hours the patch will be removed and the underlying skin examined. The skin will be checked again after ninety-six hours. If the skin is red, slightly swollen and/ or itchy, the test is considered to be positive and the material on the patch is one that is likely to cause you dermatitis when you next come into contact with it.

These tests are generally carried out while you are an outpatient and because of the times involved between examining patches you will have to be able to attend the clinic on three separate occasions in the course of one week. I know this is time-consuming, but it is very well worth while.

Besides testing the suspected material, a group of about twenty other substances that regularly cause trouble are also tested. They have been selected after intensive studies in Europe by specialists in contact dermatitis and include nickel, chromium and rubber. Similar groups of materials have been assembled in North America, chosen by the North American Contact Dermatitis Group. In this way it is possible to identify not only the material thought to be the likely cause of the trouble, but also other unsuspected materials which could cause future trouble. Smaller groups of test materials are also available for special problems – for example, a set of substances used in the manufacture of footwear for those who have problems only on their feet.

In addition to using the specially prepared tests, your dermato-logist may think it necessary to use a suitable preparation of a substance you handle regularly at work or in the course of one of your hobbies, which is why it is important to give as full a history as possible of the materials you touch, and where. Your dermato-logist will prepare a suitable dilution of the material for the test.

Patch testing looks deceptively simple but don't be tempted to try it for yourself using material you think is the trouble-maker. Things can go wrong, as I said in the last chapter. Also, you could get both false positive and false negative results because you're not using the

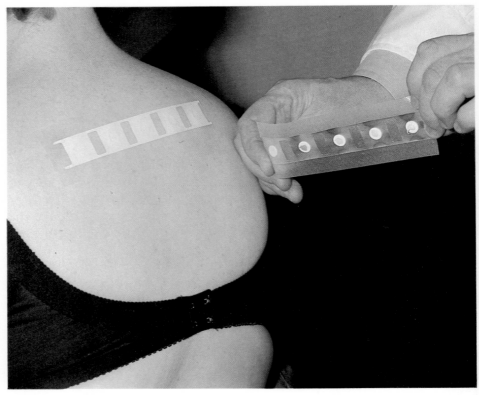

A patch test being applied.

correct concentrations, or solutions. Accurate and reliable patch tests are important and should be left to the experts.

Once these patch tests have been performed and you have been told which substances you have developed sensitivity or allergy to, your real work begins. You will most probably be given a list of everyday materials or objects that contain these substances. It will be relatively easy to avoid a potted primula – if that's what is causing the dermatitis – but if you are unlucky enough to have nickel dermatitis, for example, it can be very difficult indeed to avoid everything containing the metal and may involve many irritating and annoying changes in your lifestyle. These, however, are going to be necessary if the appearance of your skin is to return to normal, and only you can reorganize your own lifestyle (see chapter six) so as to avoid the sensitizers and the everyday objects in which they are found.

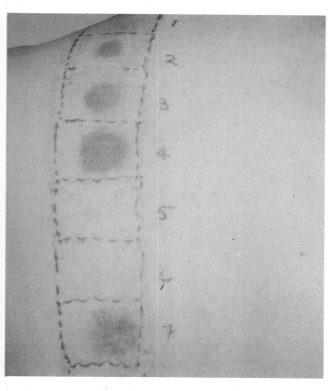

The skin's reaction to the different materials in a patch test.

Other specialized tests

From time to time other more specialized tests may also be needed. You could, for instance, need a range of tests to investigate what might be suspected to be a rare form of dermatitis caused or aggravated by natural sunlight – photosensitivity dermatitis. If these or other studies are considered necessary in your case, they will be fully explained to you.

Tests, however, are just the beginning of your cure – or at least, relief from the more unpleasant effects of your dermatitis. Armed with the results of these, you can now begin the treatment, which we shall consider in the next chapter.

5 TREATMENTS

Even though dermatitis is divided into several types, treatment is generally designed to heal or alleviate the stages most types go through. Different preparations will be advised for you when it is at the acute stage of red rash and small blisters, perhaps another at the weeping stage, something else to remove or soften the crusted stage, another at the scaly stage and yet another to deal with the abnormally thickened – or lichenified – skin.

There is a whole battery of preparations to suit different stages – lotions and creams for acute and subacute, and thicker ointments and pastes for the chronic stage, for example. Again, treatment will differ according to your reactions to particular forms of treatment. Your treatment will be prescribed especially for you and should never be handed on to anyone else. Obviously, then, the observations in this chapter will be in the nature of generalized and commonsense points that will help all dermatitis sufferers.

How, where and when to use it

Skin specialists nowadays have a wide range of treatments that will improve dermatitis. It would be overoptimistic to promise that it is possible to produce totally normal skin in every case, but most people can be made much more comfortable with regular use of creams or ointments and also possibly pills or syrups. The essential points with all of these preparations are:

1. Follow your doctor's instructions about how much to use and how often. Some creams should be applied very sparingly. Other pastes or ointments should be thickly applied.
2. Use only those preparations prescribed for your own condition. A cream that has worked wonders for a relative or neighbour could be useless or even harmful on your skin. This is particularly important in the case of children. What may start out as a slight rash in a single place may, with the wrong preparation, turn into a chronic condition.

3. Remember that in many chronic conditions, such as certain varieties of dermatitis, there are two phases of treatment. The first is treating an acute flare up, and the second is keeping the condition at bay – maintenance treatment. The more conscientiously maintenance treatment is carried out the less often will it be necessary to treat the acute flare up.

4. It goes without saying that you will keep all your preparations – especially the pills and syrups – out of the reach of children.

Creams, lotions, ointments and pastes

Preparations containing steroids (cortisone)

Most people suffering from dermatitis will have had a prescription for one of the topical steroid or cortisone-containing preparations. These have now been in use for more than twenty years and are one of the most important advances made in treating dermatitis this century.

The preparations have an anti-inflammatory effect on skin which is red, scaly, moist and sore. The cells from the bloodstream (lymphocytes and neutrophils) which have helped to cause the redness and soreness tend to move away from the skin treated with these creams and so the itch is less troublesome.

Properly used they are extremely helpful, but like all powerful forms of treatment they carry the risk of possible side-effects, particularly if used over large areas of skin on a young child, or on the thin skin of your face. Signs that your skin has had an overdose of one of these creams include the development of small visible blood vessels on your skin, and stretch marks – as seen in pregnancy – in your body folds.

Nowadays these cortisone-containing creams can be divided into four main groups:

1. **Weak**   such as Hydrocortisone.
2. **Medium**   such as Locoid, Eumovate and Haelan.
3. **Strong**   such as Synalar, Propaderm, Betnovate and Valisone.
4. **Very strong**   such as Dermovate and Synalar forte.

Your doctor will decide which strength is needed for your skin but if a strong preparation is required, he may well try to switch to a milder preparation at the next visit. Most doctors will try to use as mild a steroid or cortisone preparation as is required to control dermatitis, which is why you may receive many changes of

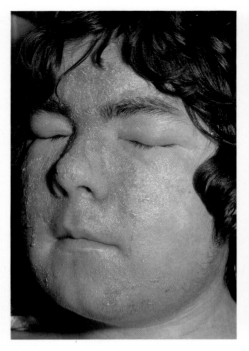
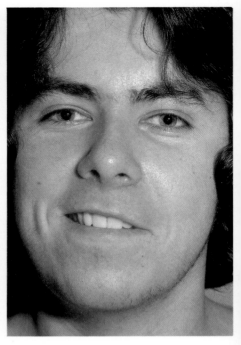

A bad case of allergic contact dermatitis before treatment.

Dramatic clearance of the skin after just five days treatment with a prescribed steroid cream.

prescription.

All steroid/cortisone prescriptions should be used sparingly and a very thin film is all that is required. Often they contain extra substances such as antibiotics to prevent or help clear additional infection – Locoid C, for example. Many of these cause a slight yellow staining of the skin. It is often necessary to use two different steroid preparations at the same time – a mild one would be prescribed for the face and a stronger one for the body. Be careful not to mix the two and use them in the wrong places.

Preparations containing tar

Grey or black creams, pastes and ointments containing tar have been used by dermatologists for more than one hundred years. Their safety is therefore well established and they are still one of the most effective forms of treatment for dermatitis, particularly in the chronic phase where the skin has become thickened and coarse. One of the effects of tar on this abnormally thickened skin is to return it to

Tar bandaging

Tar bandaging is good for most types of dermatitis, particularly when in the chronic stage. This sequence shows a tar bandage being applied to varicose dermatitis. The bandage may be left on for up to a week and renewed by the patient once he or she has been shown how to do so by a nurse.

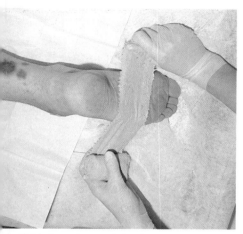

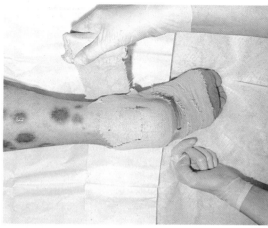

1. With leg elevated, begin to unwind the tar bandage around the foot. A protective sheet and thin plastic or rubber gloves will help to prevent mess.

2. Continue bandaging firmly around the ankle and up the leg.

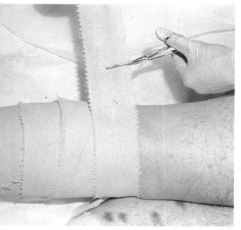

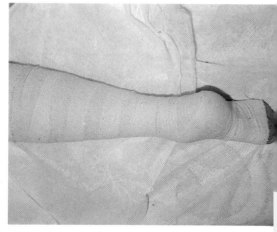

3. Finish bandaging just below the knee and secure the end with safety pins.

4. To protect clothing from staining, a crepe bandage is applied to cover the tar bandage completely.

normal, and in dermatitis generally it has an antiseptic healing and soothing effect.

Tar preparations are best used under a dressing bandaged in place. This bandage will have the additional advantage in the case of children of preventing scratching and rubbing – both of which are important causes of dermatitis failing to settle down. Most tar preparations are dispensed in tins or jars but Meditar stick comes with a twist-up stick applicator.

You will get some greyish black staining on your clothes where they come into contact with the tar. This is unavoidable unless you can shield your clothes from it in some way. Bandaging will help, so will an old vest or pyjama trousers used under your outdoor clothing if it is necessary to use the tar preparations by day as well as by night.

Sticky, tar-impregnated bandages such as Coltapaste or Tarband may be applied to the dermatitis of your legs (arms, too, occasionally) and left on the skin for several days at a time. They may be inconvenient – it is not possible to bath or shower while they are in position – but the smooth, normal skin seen when they are removed will make the temporary inconvenience well worth while.

Side-effects from tar are very rare, though some patients develop

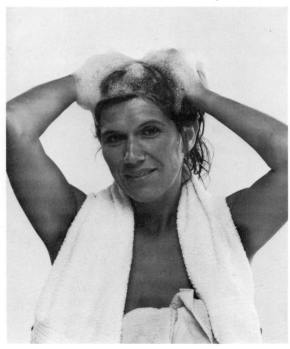

Dermatitis of the scalp can be improved by using a shampoo containing tar.

boils on hairy areas of the body, such as the lower parts of the legs.

If you have dermatitis of the scalp, you may be prescribed a tar-containing shampoo or scalp application. It is important that you leave it in contact with your scalp for a reasonable period of time if you're to obtain any benefit. Your doctor will advise you how long, and how often to use it.

Ichthyol preparations

Pastes, ointments and bandages containing ichthyol or ichthammol are also of great value in healing the skin of the dermatitis sufferer. They are often used in place of tar and are slightly cleaner but less useful if skin is very thickened. Some dermatologists suggest the use of ichthammol pastes on top of a thin layer of steroid ointment. This 'sandwich' can be a very effective treatment as well as ensuring that the steroid preparation stays in contact with your skin rather than being rubbed off on clothes or sheets.

Emollients and moisture-retaining preparations

Many dermatitis patients – especially those with the irritant contact variety – have dry skin. This in itself can cause itch and irritation, as most of us have experienced during the dryness and peeling that follows sunburn. Your doctor may suggest controlling your dry skin by the regular use of bath oils and creams which will help the skin retain moisture, and your dermatitis may be very much less troublesome. An important added bonus is of course that this means less need for the steroid-containing preparations previously described.

There are a large number of excellent emollients and dry-skin preparations: some will be prescribed by your doctor, others can be bought in any chemist or pharmacy. Only trial and error will decide which is best for your skin. Some names for British sufferers are Aquadrate, Calmurid, Oilatum emollient, Natuderm, Boots E45 cream, Unguentum Merck, Aqueous Cream BP and emulsifying ointment BP. In North America, Purpose, Jergens, Alpha-Keri and Nutraderm are all widely available; and in Australia, Aquacare and Dermafilm. As soap has a drying effect on skin, the use of an emulsifying ointment instead of soap on children's skin can make bath time much less of an ordeal.

Once again make sure you know how and when to apply these lubricants. Some should be added to the bath (it's a good idea to use a non-slip mat in the bath as it may become very slippy!), others should be rubbed gently into wet skin after the bath, and others are for use throughout the day after washing hands.

Bandages and dressings

The cream, ointment or paste your doctor prescribes for your dermatitis is an important step towards improving the condition of your skin. These preparations can, however, be very much more effective if they are properly held in position on your skin. Some preparations should be rubbed gently into the skin and left uncovered. Others should be applied under a dressing. It will depend on the type and severity of your dermatitis, and to some extent on your environment, so when your doctor gives you a prescription be sure you understand how he wants you to apply it: how often it should be changed, how to clean off the old cream and so on.

For dermatitis on the face the usual policy is for anyone treating themselves at home to use the cream alone with no covering dressing. This rule will probably not apply to a child admitted to the hospital for intensive treatment. The treatment is usually a face mask held in place with elasticated dressings, which often speeds up the healing process.

For dermatitis on other parts of the body you will almost certainly be advised to put a bandage over a dressing after applying the ointment or paste. This has a double purpose. First, it keeps the preparation on the affected area. Second, it protects your clothes and bedding from the staining that unfortunately accompanies some of the most effective treatments. An ideal method is to obtain strips of old sheets – linen if possible – and apply the thick tar or ichthyol pastes to those with a flat knife, just like spreading butter on bread. This is then laid on the inflamed skin and bandaged in place.

For hands and feet the most practical dressings are cotton gloves and socks. These can be taped on overnight to help prevent scratching.

For varicose dermatitis you may need specialized forms of bandaging to help prevent fluid accumulating around your ankles and to help the circulation in your legs – perhaps something like a blue line bandage or Bisgaard bandaging. If you do require either of these, you will be given them – and possibly help and advice on putting them on from a district nurse.

The choice of bandages is important. The elasticated gauze dressings supplied in tube form are very effective but prescribing rules vary as to whether or not these can be obtained from your family

How to put on a firm support (blue line) bandage for varicose dermatitis

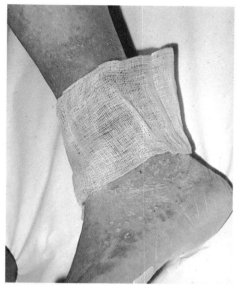

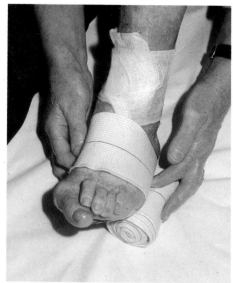

1. Protect the area of broken skin with a soft dressing or surgical gauze.

2. Firmly apply bandage, starting at the foot, which should be elevated, and continue to unwind upwards.

3. Wind bandage tightly round your leg, but not tight enough to pinch the skin.

4. Secure the top of the bandage with a couple of safety pins.

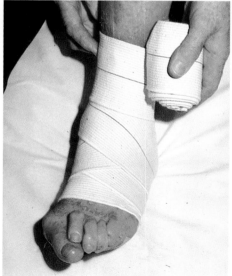

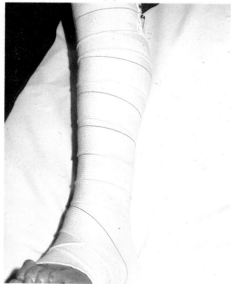

doctor on prescription. At the time of writing some widths of these dressings can be prescribed in this way and some can not.

Pills, syrups and injections

At present, the commonest prescriptions for preparations to be taken by mouth are for antihistamines and antibiotics.

Antihistamines

These are used because of their anti-itch properties. They act against the histamine liberated in the skin by cells involved in the dermatitis reaction. Histamine stimulates the desire to scratch and once the scratching habit is begun, a cycle of itch, provoking more scratching, provoking more itch, develops. This is difficult to halt, particularly in children, who very quickly develop the scratching habit if they are bored, tired or tense. Antihistamines will help reduce the itch and the need to scratch, and are particularly useful when you want a good night's sleep free of discomfort.

There are many different antihistamine pills and syrups available such as trimeprazine (Vallergan), promethazine (Phenergan), chlorpheniramine (Piriton), and as with the steroid ointments your doctor will change prescriptions until he finds the preparation most suitable for your treatment. An important point here is that the body – a child's especially – appears to adjust to many of these pills and syrups and larger doses are required as time goes by to produce the same effect. This is one of the reasons for frequent changes in the antihistamine syrup prescribed.

Many antihistamine preparations make you drowsy or sleepy, so use them with caution if you drive vehicles or operate machinery at work. Your doctor will advise you of any possible problems due to your antihistamine. To be effective, antihistamines must be given by mouth, or, very rarely, by injection. Antihistamines applied to the skin in an ointment or cream are not so effective and, indeed, may actually cause dermatitis.

Antibiotics

One hazard of dermatitis is that it is easier to develop a skin infection, particularly with the chronic atopic dermatitis of childhood. Infection greatly slows down healing as well as causing pain and swelling in addition to itch. Although doctors commonly prescribe steroid ointments with additional anti-infective agents to try to reduce the likelihood of infection, this is not always enough, and a course of antibiotics given by mouth may be necessary. This is usually given as a five-to-seven-day course of syrup or capsules. These must be taken until the course is finished, not just until the skin looks better. This is important because if you do not do this you will find that next time they will not be as effective.

Other preparations by mouth or injection
Very occasionally, and only in very severe cases of dermatitis, it may be necessary to give corticosteroid preparations by mouth or by injection for short periods of time. These have the same anti-inflammatory action as the steroids described earlier in the chapter.

One of the possible side-effects of these pills in adults is that they can reduce your ability to cope with stress. So if you have to take one of these preparations by mouth you should carry a special blue 'steroid card' so that adjustments to the dose can be made during a period of stress such as an operation for something unrelated to dermatitis. It would also be wise to let your dentist know that you are taking steroid pills if any major dental procedures are planned.

Artificial sunlight treatment

Sometimes dermatitis improves in sunny weather. If this is the case with you, your specialist may well prescribe a course of suitable artificial sunlight during the winter months. Although an easy and pleasant form of treatment, it will benefit only a small number of people. Don't rush into it by yourself – it can also have a harmful effect on skin, causing premature ageing, wrinkling and sagging of the tissues underneath the skin surface. The skin of older people is always more sensitive to sunlight, and dries out very easily – don't speed the process up! You will have your course of ultraviolet light prescribed for you, if you need it. Don't use a sun lamp at home without supervision; it can be hazardous and could cause burning of the skin and eye damage.

Supervision of dermatitis treatment

Patients with chronic dermatitis can have their treatment supervised either by their family doctor or by specialist dermatologists. Nowadays many family doctors have a particular interest and expertise in a specialist subject – diabetes, for example, skin disease or the care of the elderly. If your doctor has an interest in dermatitis – and most family doctors see a great deal of this condition, particularly in children – he will probably want to supervise your treatment himself, sending only particularly puzzling or difficult cases to the specialist.

If you are recommended to see a specialist it will usually be because your dermatitis is particularly acute, or very slow to respond to treatment, or because you require patch testing. Occasionally, there may be some doubt over the exact diagnosis, and a skin biopsy will be needed to clarify the problem. The next step will depend upon where you live, of course, and I must emphasize that the kind of routine I'm describing here is what is found generally in Britain and other countries with a state-run health service. In some countries the situation may be quite different. In the United States, for instance, there are dermatologists in general practice and if a second opinion, or even more expert advice is required, there are dermatitis specialists who can be consulted.

Waiting lists for specialist state-funded skin clinics vary considerably and if your family doctor knows the waiting list is long he may not wish to advise you to see the specialist as he knows there will be a three to four month delay, at the end of which time your skin may be quite clear anyway. The opposite situation may also apply and if your doctor knows that there is a local specialist with a short waiting list and a particular interest in dermatitis, you may get an early consultation.

You may be asked by your local specialist if you would like to take part in a trial of a new treatment for dermatitis. This is always voluntary and no one will worry if you say 'no'. Remember, however, that these trials are the best way of finding out about new treatment and no doctor will ever use anything that could be harmful. All plans for these trials must be specially approved by local committees before you are even approached and the worst that could happen is that the treatment could be less effective than was hoped. Studies on animals or on skin grown in a test-tube are much less valuable so we all hope that some of you will be willing to take part in such trials, and thereby help all dermatitis sufferers.

The important point to remember is that both family doctors and dermatologists have access to the same methods of treatment. As new methods of treatment become available, details are published in the medical journals that are read by most members of the medical profession, so there is very little risk of your family doctor not being aware of an important breakthrough or advance in treatment.

Remember also that you are the most important operator as far as treatment is concerned. Once you have been given the necessary creams and ointments it is up to you to use them according to the directions you were given – and again I emphasize, do make quite sure you know exactly how, when, and where to apply these preparations before leaving the doctor. The routine of applying these creams is time-consuming and you may be tempted to miss treatments. If you do, your skin is likely to become more irritable, and this is an excellent sign that your treatment is effective – and that perseverance is essential.

In general, very few people with dermatitis require admission to the hospital, and again this will vary in some countries according to the length of waiting lists. Although many people find their dermatitis will clear very rapidly while in the hospital, a great many find that it all comes back again when they go home. In the long run, it is really better to learn how to live with your dermatitis and how to manage it in your own home.

6 LIVING WITH DERMATITIS

What you can do to help your child and yourself

There is a tendency for anyone with a long-term illness to become discouraged and depressed by the need for regular treatment and this can be particularly true of skin disease. Regular treatment, as I have said, is time-consuming and can be messy. Healthy, normal-looking skin is an important part of normal physical attractiveness and even minor skin problems can lead to tremendous self-consciousness and loss of confidence. This is particularly true for teenagers where even those with totally normal skin go through phases of shyness and self-consciousness. Younger children starting school for the first time can also suddenly become very aware of their unsightly or peculiar skin because of the remarks – actually more thoughtless than unkind – made by their new classmates. This can quite naturally lead to a reluctance to take part in normal activities such as gymnastics, swimming and even general socializing.

If your child is gently prepared for possible questions about his skin he will find it easier to cope with the problems that will arise. Encourage him to answer in a straightforward manner – something along the lines of 'some people have upset skin just like others have upset tummies or bad headaches, and it's not catching.'

Obviously, teachers and play-leaders need to know about atopic dermatitis as their attitude can be of tremendous value in helping both your child and the other children to develop a natural, matter-of-fact approach to the problem. The most valuable thing that you as a parent can provide over this period and over all other periods of stress in your child's life is a calm, relaxed, confident home environment – not an easy task if your child's dermatitis is causing everyone sleepless nights, or at an older age, creating problems with finding a first job. It is a well-recognized fact, though, that tension and anxiety can bring on an attack of dermatitis or cause a skin inflammation that is healing to flare up again.

Coping with itch

While shyness and self-consciousness are two of the main psychological problems for the young dermatitis sufferer, itch is certainly one of the most important physical ones. Not only can it be irritating and distressing itself, but it leads, as I have said, to the vicious circle of itch/scratch/itch that will result in the aggravation of your child's dermatitis, and possibly in infection.

It is not possible to give parents definitive step-by-step instructions that are guaranteed to alleviate this problem, as each child will respond differently to whatever is done to help; and in any case itch is very difficult to get rid of completely. You should find out what works best by trial and error. Here are a few suggestions you might find useful:

1. Conscientiously carry out the treatment your doctor has prescribed. Many preparations, as we have seen, are specifically used to combat itch.
2. Try to provide as calm an atmosphere at home as possible.
3. Explain to your child if he or she is old enough, that scratching makes the itching worse rather than better.
4. Boredom is almost certain to lead to scratching, so aim to keep your child entertained for as much of the day as you can. This is bound to be exhausting for you, so try to involve the rest of the family in this whenever they are at home.
5. Itch is likely to get worse when a child is overtired and fretful. Reading a bedtime story is a good way of taking his mind off the tingling of his skin and may well send him quickly to sleep.
6. Avoid extremes of temperature. If your child is too hot or too cold his desire to scratch will increase. Watch the temperature of the bath too, as hot water will have the same effect.
7. A tepid bath with the following additives helps to soothe itchy skin: Aveeno oatmeal bath (oilated) or Emulsiderm, or Oilatum.
8. Make sure your baby or child is dressed in suitable clothing (see page 78).
9. Keep your child's fingernails short and clean.

What can be done to make the home a safer place for the dermatitis sufferer?

Over the years doctors have reported that sometimes people with chronic dermatitis experience a dramatic clearance of their skin when they move to a different part of the country. Obviously, very few people are in a position to move just to clear their dermatitis and in

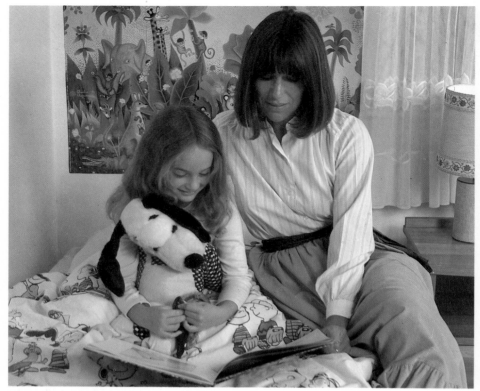

Reading a bedtime story will help relax your child and take her mind off her itching skin.

any case a cure is not guaranteed. In general, though, a mild dry climate at a high altitude in the mountains is associated with fewer cases of chronic atopic dermatitis than a humid environment. Short of moving to another part of the country there are many things that can be done to make life in the home less uncomfortable for the atopic dermatitis sufferer.

Family pets are really not to be recommended, as both cat and dog hair can aggravate atopic dermatitis. Smaller furry animals may also cause trouble. For the real enthusiast a bowl of goldfish would appear to be harmless and can even soothe frayed nerves!

Caged birds are not a good idea, though. Feathers should be avoided, especially by those who have both dermatitis and asthma. Pillows, cushions and Continental quilts or duvets should, therefore, be filled with synthetic fibre rather than natural feathers or down.

74

Dust in the house should be kept to a minimum if you have someone suffering from atopic dermatitis, though it's not an easy task. In general, carpets and curtains or drapes and loose fabric furnishings tend to attract and retain dust. So go for hard flooring surfaces such as linoleum or vinyl, blinds, and chairs without soft fabric covers, especially in the sufferer's bedroom.

Heat Almost anyone with dermatitis is more comfortable in a cool rather than a very warm environment. Try turning down the central-heating thermostat a few degrees, it could make a big difference to the itchiness. Other family members can wear an extra sweater, and everyone will benefit from the lower fuel bills!

House plants should be chosen with care. The plant most commonly associated with allergic contact dermatitis is the primula obconica, but chrysanthemums, geraniums, cineraria and other flowering plants may also cause problems.

If there is any suspicion that the dermatitis is being worsened by a plant, remove it and watch carefully for any improvement in the condition of your skin. Many hay fever sufferers are happier without indoor plants and flowers.

Drying and abrasive materials It is not uncommon for pre-school children with atopic dermatitis to develop dryness and hacking on their hands after handling chalks or sand or water. All of these are drying and abrasive and can further irritate already sensitive and inflamed skin. Alternative activities using paints, felt-tip pens and other materials can easily be arranged.

Food and the child with dermatitis

Many mothers want to know if their child with atopic dermatitis should be on a special diet or should avoid certain foods. The complicated arguments at present going on between doctors about the relationship between foods and atopic dermatitis suggests that there is not an easy or straightforward answer to this question.

Much research is at present going on into the relationship between diet in the very early months of life and the later development of dermatitis. Ten years ago it was suggested that children who were exclusively breast fed from birth were less likely to develop atopic dermatitis than those who received supplementary bottle feeds or were exclusively bottle fed. This led many doctors to advise those mothers with a family history of atopic dermatitis to breast feed their

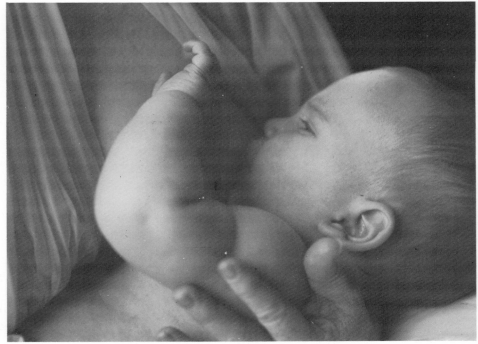

If you have a strong family history of atopic dermatitis it is advisable to breast feed your baby.

baby for at least six months with absolutely no supplementary bottle feeds, and also to delay the introduction of mixed feeding. In some cases this appears to have been successful, and in spite of strong family histories of atopic dermatitis the babies have not had any problems. On the other hand, others treated in this way have still developed dermatitis.

We still need to know more about the exact relationship between food protein absorbed from the gut and the skin rash before confident advice on infant feeding can be given. That doesn't mean, of course, that we can't draw up a few points on feeding your baby, and some sensible attitudes to diet and your child with atopic dermatitis. In general:

1. Breast feed your baby if possible if you have a strong family history of atopic dermatitis, and allow no supplementary cow's milk feeds. Breast feeding may not prevent dermatitis, but could cut down the numbers of children who develop dermatitis and the severity of the condition in others.

2. Wean later rather than earlier.

3. Watch carefully reactions to cow's milk, eggs (yolk and white separately) and fish. These three protein foods are the ones that most commonly cause problems in young children with atopic dermatitis. Swelling or itching of the lips may occur within minutes of eating the food, and pain or sickness may occur from one to two hours later. It is difficult to be sure that these examples of food intolerance lead directly to a flare up of the rash as this may not happen until between one and two days later.

Some children can take egg yolks safely, others egg white; an egg-yolk custard will contain one, and meringues the other. Try each of these at different times and watch carefully for any reaction.

4. If you find that your child reacts to a large number of protein foods seek medical advice. All young children need adequate amounts of protein for healthy growth and development. It is these protein foods that may cause problems in young children with dermatitis and advice from a qualified dietician will be valuable.

5. If you think your child is allergic to cow's milk, possible alternatives are goat's milk or milk made from soya protein (Prosobee, for example). A study on a small number of atopic dermatitis sufferers who were given soya protein in place of other essential dairy proteins for a short period suggests that when dairy proteins – milk, cheese and so on – are removed from the diet and this vegetable protein is substituted there was an improvement in the dermatitis. Not for all, unfortunately. Obviously a great deal more research is needed.

Both soya protein and goat's milk provide much of the essential daily protein, but these special diets need the full co-operation of your child, and are particularly difficult to organize if your child has reached school age.

6. In general, food intolerance tends to improve as your child gets older. A young child who reacts to several foods may sometimes appear to exist on a very limited and dull range of food. Remember that even children with perfectly normal skin can be very fussy and faddy over food at this age. Every two or three months try to reintroduce one of the foods that previously caused problems.

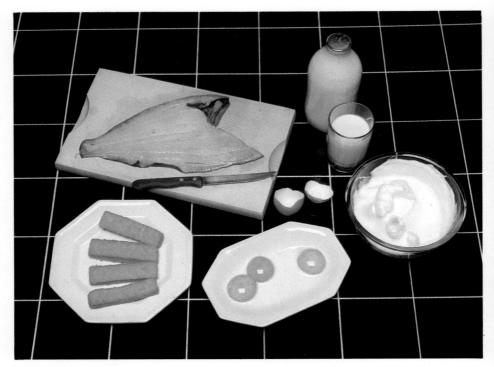

Children with atopic dermatitis often react badly to protein foods such as fish, milk and eggs. Some may be allergic just to egg yolk, others to egg white.

Offer just a small spoonful at first and observe the result. By the age of five or six years most children will have outgrown the food-related problems that were present at the age of one to two years.

7. For older children, a normal varied diet is recommended. Until we understand better the relationship between the foods we eat and atopic dermatitis there is no need to prepare special meals for the atopic child unless this is suggested by your doctor or specialist.

Clothing

Cotton In general, pure cotton is the best material for clothing next to the skin of someone with atopic dermatitis. Wool, nylon and other synthetic fibres can irritate the skin, so use them only as outer layers and watch for contact at areas such as the wrist and neckline.

Pure cotton can be difficult to find as too many materials nowadays are of mixed fibres, mainly synthetic with just a small proportion of cotton. Those living in North America are more fortunate than those living in Britain as pure cotton clothing is more easily available there. In Britain the National Eczema Society has been encouraging manufacturers to provide pure cotton clothing, particularly for children, and your local branch of the Society may be able to send you a list of suppliers. For older children and adults, sporting goods stores may be helpful, particularly for cotton socks.

Covering up To help prevent scratching, babies with itchy dermatitis should be dressed in stretch-suits that cover feet and hands; and young children should wear clothes that cover and protect the skin without being tight or restricting. Girls will be more comfortable in cotton tights or trousers and boys in long trousers. It is important not to put on too many layers of clothing because overheating is a common cause of triggering off a bout of scratching. Speak to your child's teacher about the kind of clothing he's most comfortable in. Schools are usually understanding if your child is comfortable in clothing that is not a regular part of a suggested uniform. For knitted

Stretch-suits that cover hands and feet will help to prevent your baby scratching.

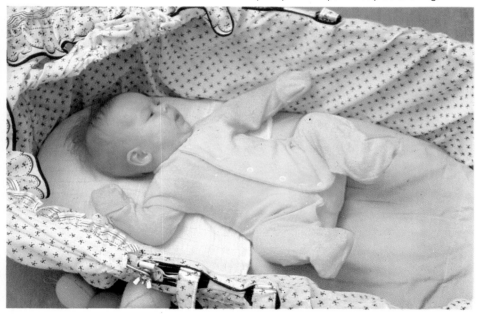

sweaters and other clothes in winter, it is better to make them from a synthetic yarn – worn over cotton underclothes – as pure wool is more likely to irritate even the small areas of contact around the neck and the wrists.

Hands that are affected by dermatitis can be particularly painful in cold damp winter weather. The skin easily becomes dry and chapped, and splits, especially around finger joints, and often becomes infected. It is wise to avoid putting hands like this in water and to use thin cotton gloves under rubber gloves when dishwashing or other household chores are essential. Young children with hand problems should be persuaded to wear gloves for all outdoor activities.

Cosmetics

Teenage girls with dermatitis will naturally want to present a good appearance to the world and may be keen to experiment with make-up, hair preparations and other aids to beauty. This experi-

If you are prone to irritant contact dermatitis, use cotton 'inners' under rubber gloves when washing up.

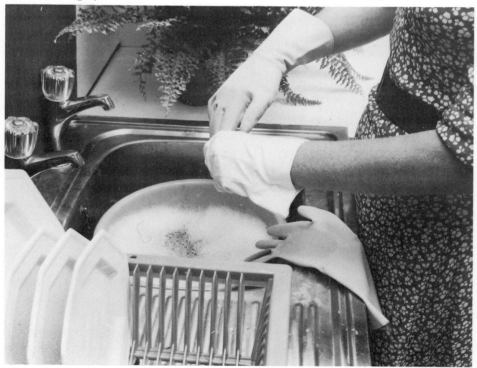

mentation is a normal part of growing up and if you have a daughter suffering from dermatitis she should be able to take part quite safely provided she takes a few simple precautions.

For the face   In general, skin affected by dermatitis is dry. There is at least one advantage of this, which is that people with dermatitis have acne less often than average, as acne tends to attack those with a greasy skin. You have to be very unfortunate to have both acne and dermatitis. Girls with dermatitis should, therefore, use cosmetics designed for a normal or dry skin rather than a greasy one.

Some dermatitis sufferers are more prone to allergies to cosmetics than average and may want to use special hypo-allergenic or fragrance-free preparations. Many of these are of high quality but are also expensive. A sensible compromise is to buy a small quantity of an inexpensive make-up and apply it to a small area of skin to see if there is any discomfort or stinging. Once you have found cosmetics that do not sting or irritate the skin it is a good idea to stick to the same brand.

Lanolin can be a cause of dermatitis in some people. Clearly they must avoid hand creams, moisture creams and the like that contain it. Excessive use of soap and water is drying and irritating to dermatitis-prone skin. There are some gentle non-soap cleansers on the market and these should be used. Liberal use of moisture creams and emollients can make a dramatic difference to dry, parched, scaling skin and such preparations are, of course, all free of the possible side-effects associated with steroid creams.

For the hands and eyes   Nail varnish and eye make-up can also irritate the dermatitis sufferer's skin and the best advice is to stick to one brand after carefully applying small amounts to your skin or nails to avoid possible trouble. Remember, though, that manufacturers can change the ingredients used in a brand of cosmetic and still package it in identical containers.

Hair
People with dermatitis often have a scaly or irritable scalp. Special shampoos containing tar and other preparations may be quite soothing, but you should leave them on your hair and scalp for a few minutes while shampooing to obtain any benefit.

Many of the hair dyes and tints available nowadays can safely be used, but dyes containing para phenylene diamine (PPD), are a well-recognized cause of allergic contact dermatitis. The letters PPD will be seen on the packet and the manufacturer's instructions give clear and sensible advice about applying a patch test before using the dye.

Even with these precautions you may still have problems, particularly with do-it-yourself dyes bought in the pharmacy to use at home. The best policy is to settle for a comfortable simple hairstyle without dyeing or permanent waves. If either of these is essential, a visit to a good hairdresser is a very much better idea than home tinting, bleaching or perming.

Jewellery

This can also be a source of trouble for anyone suffering from dermatitis. Those sensitive to nickel will find that nearly all inexpensive metal jewellery contains some nickel and must be avoided. If you are not sure about the nickel content a clear fluid solution can be bought, which, when painted on the metal (a watchstrap, say, or earrings), will become pink if nickel is present. This is a very useful

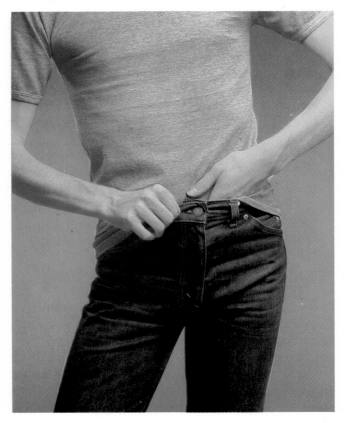

'Jean-stud' nickel dermatitis can be prevented simply by wearing your tee-shirt tucked in at the waist.

82

and sensible way of preventing trouble. Your own doctor or dermatologist can tell you where this fluid can be obtained.

A common site of trouble in young people who are nickel-sensitive is a patch of skin on their stomachs. This is due to the nickel button on their denim jeans. Twenty years ago 'jean-stud' nickel dermatitis was unheard of, but now with changing fashions and the universal teenage uniform of jeans, it is quite a common problem. It is easily avoided by wearing a cotton tee-shirt tucked in at the waistband.

Careers – choices and pitfalls

Even though the world is in a recession and jobs are hard to find, it is still important for all young people to look for a career they will enjoy and which will not create health problems. The teenager with dermatitis appears to be doubly hampered, for at a time of serious teenage unemployment the temptation to take any job that's offered is strong, but we still have to advise him or her to avoid certain types of work. For we know from long experience that certain occupations are likely to be associated with flare ups of the condition, spells off work and eventually disappointment and loss of confidence at having to leave the job. In these circumstances, training in a new skill can be provided, but how much better it is to settle in the first place for a job that is unlikely to provoke skin problems.

Two careers to avoid are nursing and hairdressing. Both involve long hours spent with your hands in water or water and detergents, and in neither is it possible to do all aspects of the job well if you're constantly wearing gloves.

Unfortunately, many youngsters with chronic atopic dermatitis have got to know well the atmosphere of a hospital and the nurses who help care for them. It is a very pleasant compliment to our nurses that these young people wish to follow their example, but experience has shown that many atopic dermatitis sufferers have to give up nursing after six or twelve months of training.

Hairdressing can also be a hazardous occupation for anyone with dermatitis. Juniors in hairdressing establishments usually spend a lot of time shampooing and this, of course, causes dryness and chapping of the hands – sometimes even in those with otherwise normal skin and no past history of dermatitis. Later on in training, the handling of permanent-wave lotions and hair dyes can again irritate the skin.

Other unsuitable occupations include being a motor mechanic or any other job where regular contact with dirt and grease means that frequent washing is essential.

The most suitable job is one that involves working indoors in a constant temperature without having to handle materials which may irritate or sensitize the skin.

Coping at work

The people most affected here are those who develop irritant contact dermatitis through working in an environment which entails chronic exposure of their skin to materials that dissolve away the protective greasy coating of their skin. The loss of this barrier leads to dry flaking skin that easily chaps, and splits, particularly in cold weather. The way is then open for minor infections to complicate the picture.

The logical step is prevention. Anyone regularly exposed to degreasing agents should be given protective clothing. In practice, this will almost always mean the use of protective rubber or vinyl gloves, as it is your hands that are by far the most common site of irritant dermatitis. When you use rubber gloves you should always wear a pair of soft cotton gloves next to your skin to absorb perspiration. If you don't the skin of your hands will be shut up in an environment like a Turkish bath, which can be almost as bad for your skin as the degreasing materials and detergents you're wearing gloves to protect it against! Cloth-lined gloves by themselves are not enough, as these quickly become damp and saturated with perspiration.

It is important to remember that all these points apply just as much to the busy housewife as to the factory worker. Many people tend to associate dermatitis, and particularly contact dermatitis, with industrial work, but a busy young mother frequently exposes the skin of her hands to harsher agents and more rapid changes in temperature than many factory employees (see page 86).

If your dermatitis develops after you've been working at your job for a number of years, and you find that you can't avoid contact with irritant materials, you should talk to your medical officer if your company has one. Often it is possible to change your job within an office or factory and this is a very good answer to the problem. In some countries there are government retraining schemes, and in Britain the Employment Medical Advisory Service (EMAS) can also be of great support. Your own family doctor or skin specialist can provide more information about this sort of service if you need it.

A brief word here about the legal aspects of developing contact dermatitis at work. Some occupations are more at risk than others in this respect, and you may feel sufficiently aggrieved at the way you have contracted this type of dermatitis that you may wish to consider a legal claim for compensation. This is a complicated matter outside the scope of this book and anyone considering this type of action should consult their family doctor and dermatologist. As a doctor, my concern here is with the health of the sufferer so that, although your claim may be successful, the relatively small financial gain will not return your skin to normal and, furthermore, the tension and worry over a legal action may make the condition very slow to settle.

Relationships

Having sore, itchy skin – or even just blotchy skin – can take up a lot of time and energy; the pain and discomfort, the time spent on treatments and trying to disguise the more obvious marks. These inevitably make the disease loom very large in the mind of the sufferer. It is hardly surprising, therefore, that many people with dermatitis become withdrawn and lonely. The best advice in such a situation is in the first place to talk to someone else with the condition. In Britain there will probably be a branch of the National Eczema Society somewhere near you (see the list of useful addresses at the end of the book). It always helps to talk things over with a fellow-sufferer.

If you're keen on sport, or even if you would like to learn one, join a club or a beginner's class. Drawing, painting, and many other leisure activities are excellent ways of making contact with others – and forgetting about those blemishes while you're so absorbed in what you're doing!

Dermatitis and sex

It's difficult to give generalized advice about intimate problems such as how to make love when one or both partners are suffering from skin disease. Dermatitis can and does affect men's and women's genital areas – a reason in contact dermatitis to avoid as far as possible douches, vaginal deodorants, contraceptive creams and talcum powders.

If you have a rash affecting the genital area that's severe enough to interfere with sexual intercourse, then do tell your doctor or skin specialist. The sooner you mention it, the quicker it can be cleared up. Don't attempt to treat it yourself. The skin of the area is thin and highly sensitive and some preparations may be too strong and will only make matters worse.

Hobbies and vacations

In general, if you have chronic dermatitis then you should avoid hobbies and household chores that involve having your hands in water. The use of turpentine and lubricating oils in home decorating and car maintenance are also two on the 'not recommended' list.

When taking a vacation in an area that's usually a lot sunnier than where you live, take great care out of doors until you find out how your skin and your dermatitis reacts to strong sunshine. Tell your doctor before you go off on a vacation in a sunny country, as some of the pills and creams commonly used by dermatitis patients react with sunlight and he may, therefore, decide to change your treatment for a short time. You will also want to take enough treatments with you to last throughout your vacation.

Dermatitis usually improves on a vacation in the sun, but a few people with atopic dermatitis find that they are very sensitive to the sun and that their skin gets worse. If this happens to you, use a strong sun barrier cream. The efficiency of these sun barrier creams, which prevent burning, is steadily improving. The recommended brands have the letters SPF (Sun Protective Factor) on them. Nowadays, most sun creams have these letters followed by a number somewhere between 3 and 20. The higher the number, the better the protection offered. For a young child, or anyone with sun-sensitive skin, choose a preparation with an SPF of 10 or more. Always follow the manufacturers' instructions about how often to apply the cream.

Dermatitis in pregnancy and early motherhood

Many women with dermatitis find that their skin improves during pregnancy – an unexpected bonus. This improvement can continue after your baby is born but there are no definite patterns. Enjoy your pregnancy and follow your doctor's advice on diet. At present, there is no evidence that special diets during pregnancy will affect the chances of your baby having dermatitis.

Irritant contact dermatitis of the hands in women often begins or gets worse after the birth of the first baby. Babies inevitably involve the mother in a greatly increased amount of contact with soap and water. If you know you have a tendency to dermatitis try to keep this to a minimum. Disposable nappies (I think Britain is one of the few countries left with non-disposable nappies/diapers!) will cut down on washing and a fully automatic washing machine is a worthwhile investment. Rinse your hands well after baby's bathtime and use hand cream liberally. A common site of trouble is under your wedding ring. This does not necessarily mean that you have become allergic to the metal of your ring; it's more likely that dried soap has lodged there. Rinse particularly carefully and if your finger is really red and sore remove the ring for a few days.

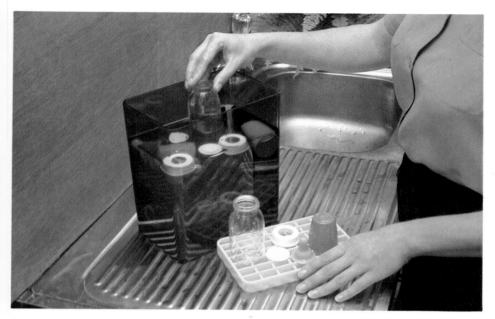

Immersing your hands frequently in bottle sterilizing solution can lead to contact dermatitis. Get in the habit of wearing rubber gloves with cotton 'inners' (see page 80).

Although water is the main culprit, dermatitis can also be triggered by contact with bottle sterilizing fluids and, if you have the non-disposable nappies/diapers, with the cleansing antiseptic solutions used to soak them in. If you find they irritate your hands try using rubber gloves – or a pair of tongs. It's surprising how adept you can be with them!

Dermatitis and other infections

Immunization and vaccinations
Preventive medicine is a most important part of child health nowadays and in developed countries most parents want their children to be protected against diseases that used to be common and sometimes fatal. Even if your baby has developed dermatitis, it is a wise precaution for it to have a course of triple vaccine against diptheria, tetanus and whooping cough (pertussis) during the first year and possibly also measles and polio immunization at around the same time.

If your child does have dermatitis and his skin is very inflamed, with new patches of the rash appearing, it is often wise to delay the injection for a week or two until the skin is quieter; but in the case of polio vaccine, which is given by mouth, there is no need to delay at all. In a few cases the child's skin may appear to flare up temporarily after his injection but this will pass. Protection against severe infectious diseases is a most important part of caring for your child in the first year of life and should not be denied to children with atopic or any other type of dermatitis.

Viral infections

Doctors and research workers have found that some people who suffer from atopic dermatitis appear to have less efficient internal defences against a few virus infections. Mumps, measles, and chickenpox cause no special problems for children with dermatitis and the viruses causing these diseases appear to be dealt with by atopic dermatitis sufferers in much the same way as by the rest of the population. The wart virus is one of those handled less efficiently, however. Although no age group is immune from them, they are more common in children and found even more often in children with atopic dermatitis than in others.

Surprisingly, it is the common cold sore that can become a serious problem to anyone with atopic dermatitis. Most of us have one infection with the virus responsible for cold sores – the herpes simplex virus – early in life and are then immune to further attacks. A few people after this first attack develop recurrent cold sores usually on the upper lip area. In people with atopic dermatitis, however, a cold sore may lead to rapid and widespread infection with the virus over the whole skin surface, and could even involve their internal organs. Because it is a serious problem, children with atopic dermatitis should be kept well away from cold sores. However tempting, mothers with cold sores should resist the comforting or goodnight kiss for their young atopic dermatitis sufferer.

A similar widespread and alarming skin eruption can develop in someone with atopic dermatitis after they've been vaccinated against smallpox, or even through being in contact with a brother or sister who has been vaccinated against smallpox. Fortunately, it is a problem very rarely seen nowadays as very few children are now vaccinated against smallpox and vaccination is no longer compulsory. Indeed, we hope that smallpox has been eradicated from the world and so this complication is becoming merely historical. In the meantime, smallpox vaccination and contact with those recently vaccinated must be avoided by all those with active atopic dermatitis and also

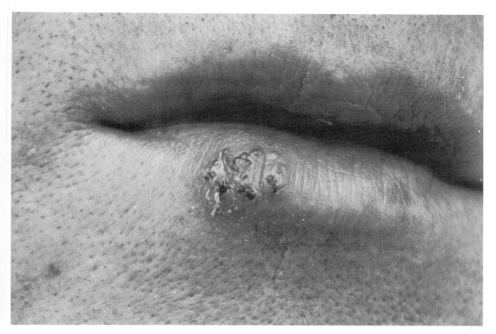

Atopic dermatitis sufferers should be kept away from anyone who has cold sores (herpes simplex).

with those who have had atopic dermatitis in the year or two previously.

Protecting your child
To sum up, then: if your child or anyone in your family suffers from atopic dermatitis remember these three important points:

1. **Do** have your child vaccinated against diphtheria, tetanus and whooping cough.
2. **Don't** let them come into contact with anyone suffering from cold sores.
3. **Don't** let them be vaccinated against smallpox and keep them well away from anyone else who has been recently vaccinated against smallpox.

7 LESS COMMON TYPES OF DERMATITIS

Even though these three types of dermatitis are rare and easily distinguishable from other forms, treatment is the same. That is, they are treated according to the stage they are at – red rash and blisters, weeping and crusted, raised areas of thickened or lichenified skin. Exfoliative or severely scaling dermatitis, the last of these rare forms, requires special medical care and should be treated in the hospital.

Nummular (discoid or coin-shaped) dermatitis

This dermatitis usually appears suddenly as coin-shaped circular areas on the skin. The commonest parts of the body to be affected are the lower arms and, more usually, the lower legs. There is no good explanation for the circular form of these lesions, and by patch testing we know that they are not due to allergy to any material. They appear most often in young adults and especially in those who in the past have had atopic dermatitis. They also appear on people who have no such history of atopic dermatitis but on the other hand may be exposed to detergents and other degreasing agents – suggesting that this may be a form of irritant contact dermatitis.

The coin-shaped areas of nummular dermatitis may vary in size. The whole surface of the circle is red and crusted and easily becomes infected. As with adult seborrhoeic dermatitis it can be a very stubborn condition and slow to clear.

Neurodermatitis or 'nervous' dermatitis

This dermatitis, with the medical name lichen simplex chronicus, occurs most commonly in middle life. It usually starts as a very severe itch which inevitably leads to scratching or rubbing of the affected area, frequently the back of the neck. As this continues for

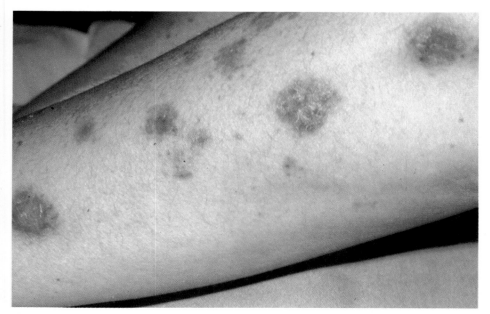

The characteristic coin shape of nummular dermatitis.

several weeks, the skin's natural response to being continually rubbed, buffed or scratched is for the number of cells in the epidermis, or outer layer, to be increased and so the skin becomes thicker, or lichenified. This shows as a raised reddish-blue patch with the normal skin creases and lines very much emphasized. Once this develops, a vicious circle sets in as the rubbing and scratching stimulate further skin thickening which in turn seems to trigger off itch within the area, which causes yet more scratching. It occurs often in people who have a tendency to be anxious and worried and appears to be a 'stress signal' which is worse at times of tension. If the person can be persuaded to stop scratching and rubbing, the skin returns to its normal state.

Exfoliative or severely scaling dermatitis

In normal skin, the outer layers are being continually shed and replaced by skin cells growing up from below. The rate of this skin shedding is quite slow, so unless it is speeded up, for example by sunburn, no obvious scaling or peeling is seen. In exfoliative dermatitis, though, the entire skin surface is being shed at a very much faster rate than normal and as the name suggests, the amount of falling scales can be likened to the falling of leaves in autumn.

There is a variety of causes that can trigger off this reaction and one of the commonest is a severe side-effect of a drug taken by mouth. Although there is a wide range of pills that can on some occasions cause exfoliative dermatitis, only a very few people who take these ever develop it. Sleeping pills, antibiotics and diuretics (which help the body to lose excess fluid) are among possible culprits but once again it must be stressed that the great majority of people who need these pills and have them prescribed by their doctor never have any such side-effects.

Another cause of exfoliative dermatitis is an acute flare of psoriasis, a common skin disease affecting about one person in fifty and which looks like raised red scaly patches on the knees, elbows and scalp. It is usually not itchy. For more information on psoriasis, I can recommend *Psoriasis* by Professor Ronald Marks, also in this Positive Health Guide series. A further cause is extreme and severe sensitivity to certain wavelengths in natural sunlight.

In the rapidly shed scales of skin are traces of essential materials such as iron and certain vitamins. Even more important is the extreme redness of the skin that commonly accompanies this scaling. This redness (called erythroderma) comes about through the swelling of very large numbers of tiny blood vessels just under the skin surface, and results in very rapid and extensive heat loss from the skin surface. If the sufferer is young and nursed in a warm environment this is easily corrected, but in older people, particularly if the room is not kept warm, the actual internal body temperature can fall rapidly and dramatically although the skin surface is red and warm. It is most important to keep this type of dermatitis under careful medical supervision. Associated also with this increase in blood flow through the skin is a tendency to develop puffy swelling (known as oedema) around the ankles, if you are standing or sitting, and around the back, if confined to bed. Fortunately, with suitable treatment, exfoliative dermatitis is usually of short duration and these distressing complications do not last for long.

8 CURRENT RESEARCH INTO THE CAUSES OF DERMATITIS

I think it is fair to say that as yet we do not fully understand the cause of many types of dermatitis. Because of this, and as many forms of dermatitis are so common, they are the subject of much interest and research in dermatology at the present time. More work, however, still needs to be done. In the past ten years several clues to solving some of the mysteries have been unravelled and this chapter will explain some of these.

Research into a disease such as dermatitis is very like a detective novel with various clues turning up. The final explanation for dermatitis depends on all these clues and pointers being put together in a logical manner so that apparently isolated and unrelated features of the condition can be linked and understood. Understanding a cause does not always bring about a cure, but it obviously makes the possibility of discovering a cure much more likely and, just as important, it allows preventive measures to be taken.

Some of the ideas in this chapter are rather more complicated than explanations in the rest of this book, but are hopefully of interest to dermatitis sufferers and their parents. It is perfectly possible, though, to understand and benefit from the other chapters in the book without reading this one.

Research into atopic dermatitis (childhood eczema)

Diet and atopic dermatitis

As we saw in chapter six, there are some associations between food intolerance and atopic dermatitis, which has led to the idea that foods may indeed in some cases be the cause of atopic dermatitis. Because there would seem to be more cases of atopic dermatitis among bottle-fed babies than breast-fed babies it has been suggested that cow's milk could be one of the foods. The possible reasons for this are complicated: it is thought that the bacteria which inhabit the intestines of normal healthy breast-fed babies and those that inhabit the intestines of bottle-fed babies are very different and have different effects on the body's defence systems.

We will undoubtedly hear more of these interesting ideas and theories, and perhaps over the next few years will have more firm information on the real relationship between diet and atopic dermatitis. In the meantime, it must be stressed again that all children require adequate quantities of protein for growth and development. Even if breast feeding is eventually shown to be of little importance in the prevention of atopic dermatitis, it is of value for many other reasons.

Heredity

It is clear that many people's atopic dermatitis is inherited. Exactly how this inheritance – or the genetic factor – causes the disease, is not clear. In some other diseases it is relatively easy to identify the gene responsible for the condition, but in atopic dermatitis it seems that several genes, rather than just one, may be involved, and that a combination of both inherited genes and some factor in the environment – nature and nurture – may be needed before the disease develops.

Studies of disease in identical twins are always helpful in unravelling this type of problem. If the inherited elements were all-important, then pairs of identical twins who have atopic dermatitis would have the disease in identical severity. In fact this is true in only about half of the pairs of twins studied, so heredity is not by itself the only all-important factor.

The body's immune system

One of the body's defence mechanisms against infection is a group of substances circulating in the blood, called the immunoglobulins (Ig). These defence proteins help to protect us against the various types of infection that are due mainly to bacteria. There are five main types of immunoglobulins: IgG, which is present in the largest quantities; IgM, which is important in the very early stages of immunity development; IgA, which is particularly important in maintaining defence against infection on mucous membranes such as the mouth lining and the inner membranes of the eye; and IgD and IgE. At present, we do not completely understand the function of IgD. The immunoglobulin which appears to be closely associated with atopic dermatitis is IgE.

We know that many other diseases have come about largely due to a lack of a naturally occurring material such as immunoglobulin. In the case of atopic dermatitis, however, the problem is associated with a tendency to manufacture not too little but too much IgE. Normally this material is found in the blood in tiny quantities. Its original function in evolution may have been to help in defence against parasite infections. In modern living conditions, parasite infections are fortunately uncommon and most of us do not appear to need our IgE, although this is by no means true in underdeveloped countries.

In atopic people there is a tendency for the body to make excessive quantities of IgE specifically directed against a large variety of materials, usually proteins, with which the body comes into contact. The most commonly identified materials against which this IgE is made are foods (fish, milk, eggs, peanuts, crab), pollens and the house-dust mite (which bears the grand name dermatophagoides pteronissinus).

A blood test called the RAST test carried out on a child with dermatitis aged one year or older can tell whether or not the total level of IgE is raised, and also exactly which materials the IgE is directed against. In most people with atopic dermatitis high levels will be found. There are always a few who don't follow the general pattern, though. A few who have only the atopic skin problems and not the asthma, for example, associated with it, may have normal levels. High levels of IgE can be found in a few skin conditions quite separate from atopic dermatitis. The great majority of raised IgE levels, however, are found in patients with atopic dermatitis and very high levels may be found in those who have both dermatitis and asthma.

Because a few of the patients examined had high levels of IgE in their blood and did not have atopic dermatitis, research workers believe that the high IgE itself is unlikely to be the actual cause of atopic dermatitis, but, that together they may be caused by the same stimulus and that there has to be a common link. We now think that this common cause is a subgroup of one of the white blood cell populations, the lymphocytes.

There are in fact two main subgroups of lymphocytes: the T lymphocytes, which are particularly valuable in defending the body against fungal and virus diseases, and the B lymphocytes which are of greater importance in defending our bodies against bacterial disease. The T lymphocytes are divided into at least two further subgroups which may either 'help' or 'suppress' the work of the B lymphocytes. Normally, IgE is made by B lymphocytes and is kept at a low level by the suppressor T lymphocytes. Some research workers have shown that in atopic dermatitis this delicate control mechanism is faulty and that the T suppressor or controlling lymphocytes are not performing their function adequately or are present in smaller numbers than usual.

This helps explain the high levels of IgE in atopic dermatitis sufferers, but there still is a vital link required to explain the relationship between the low levels of T suppressor lymphocytes and the actual activity of the dermatitis, and it is in this area that work is still going on.

Many people with atopic dermatitis have a very pale skin. When it is rubbed fiercely or scratched, it develops a raised white weal instead of the more usual red weal. This has led to the suggestion that in atopic dermatitis one of the chemical messengers in the bloodstream, responsible for controlling tension and tone in normal blood vessels, is defective. More research will be needed to investigate this idea further and to link it to some of the observations on lymphocytes and IgE control I have just mentioned.

Defect of the thymus gland

It is important to remember that the cells that make up the skin are not stationary objects sitting on the body surface for a lifetime. They are being continually shed at the skin surface and new cells are constantly manufactured in the deeper parts of the skin to balance this loss. In addition, the many cells present in the bloodstream circulate regularly and continuously through the lower layer of the skin, the dermis.

One of the types of white blood cells, the lymphocyte, is, as we have already seen, of possible importance in the cause of atopic dermatitis. A specialized gland behind the breast bone, the thymus gland, is important in the development of normal lymphocytes while the unborn child is developing in the womb. After birth, this thymus gland is no longer important or even necessary for this function, but a baby born with no thymus has a poorly developed lymphocyte system and is likely to develop infections.

Some research workers believe that in atopic dermatitis the affected children have a poorly functioning thymus which has not been able to mature the baby's lymphocytes in the womb. It is now possible to prepare extracts of thymus gland and to manufacture material which is very similar to the naturally occuring thymus hormones. Trials of the use of these substances in children with atopic dermatitis are already in progress and the results will be of great interest. (This is, of course, a very new development and not a treatment that can yet be prescribed by your family doctor or skin specialist.)

There are, as you can see, many theories and a few facts about the cause of atopic dermatitis. This and other allergic conditions urgently require more research to investigate these ideas further so that new hope can be brought to the very large number of sufferers.

Research into contact dermatitis

Just as with atopic dermatitis, we have in contact dermatitis a most important and relatively neglected field of research. Here we have the problem not only of suffering and discomfort but also of very significant loss of time from work leading to loss of output. It is very difficult to calculate the cost to a country of a condition such as contact dermatitis but in Britain alone it must amount to many millions of pounds annually. Clearly, therefore, a small investment of research funds is worth while to try to prevent at least some of this loss of output and associated discomfort.

Irritant contact dermatitis
Once dry chapped skin has developed, it becomes an urgent matter to replace the skin's naturally produced lubricant. Here, the pharmaceutical companies have in the past decade or so worked very closely with dermatologists to produce effective emollient creams and ointments. The results of this co-operation are impressive, and many lubricating preparations are now available that will rapidly replace moisture and oils in dry damaged skin (see page 65). These preparations are now relatively non-greasy and cosmetically very acceptable in comparison with older preparations. They have benefited not just those suffering from irritant contact dermatitis but also those with other types of dermatitis and some quite unrelated skin diseases.

An important way of preventing irritant contact dermatitis would be to increase our knowledge about the way in which the different layers of the epidermis − the outermost layers of skin − contribute to the waterproofing or barrier function of normal healthy skin. Better understanding of this could lead to the development of ways of increasing or improving the barrier function, which would obviously be extremely valuable, particularly when working with materials that require fine finger co-ordination and are too delicate to allow the use of thick protective gloves. Research of this nature is really in its infancy and more work is urgently required.

Allergic contact dermatitis

One of the fascinating problems about this particular type of dermatitis is that a material such as nickel can be handled safely and with no ill effects by 95 per cent of the population but can cause severe dermatitis in the remaining 5 per cent if they handle it. Furthermore, there's the well-recognized fact that many people handle materials such as nickel with no ill effects for many years and then suddenly, for no obvious reason, develop allergic contact dermatitis. Why are some people especially at risk, and what changes in lifestyle can cause this form of dermatitis to develop?

If we could find a way of identifying those who are at risk of developing allergic contact dermatitis, it would obviously be an important step forward. It would then be possible to ensure that they were not exposed to working conditions or to an environment in which the material causing the allergy is present. All new employees could be given a simple test and those who showed a likelihood of future allergic reaction to something in their intended workplace could be employed handling other materials or issued with appropriate protective clothing. At the moment, a way of identifying in advance those likely to develop allergic contact dermatitis is still to be developed.

Two possible methods of approach will be:

1. The development of a simple blood test designed to identify the subgroup of white blood cells, the lymphocytes, which are known to carry the 'memory' of contact with a particular material, and to multiply rapidly into an army of defending cells when the body next comes into contact with that substance.

2. A test on the skin itself: either a more sophisticated form of the commonly used patch test, or a test on a small piece of skin cut from the body (a biopsy) to examine the specialized cells – called the Langerhan's cells – involved in receiving materials absorbed through the skin and then bringing them into contact with the lymphocytes in the bloodstream.

The Langerhans' cells are shaped rather like an octopus with a central body and a number of tentacles reaching out among the other cells. The tentacles of one Langerhans' cell reach to the tentacles of similar neighbouring Langerhans' cells, forming a very efficient network or

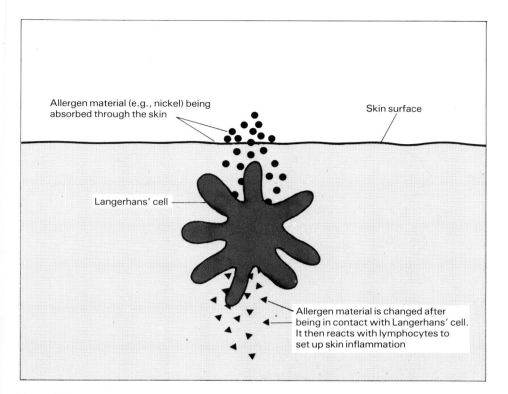

Allergen material (e.g., nickel) being absorbed through the skin

Skin surface

Langerhans' cell

Allergen material is changed after being in contact with Langerhans' cell. It then reacts with lymphocytes to set up skin inflammation

Shaped like an octopus, the Langerhans' cells play a crucial part in the contact dermatitis reaction. Researchers believe that in the future these cells – and hence contact dermatitis – may be able to be manipulated with ultraviolet light.

trap on the skin surface to gather material absorbed through the skin.

As a result of work carried out in the past ten years we know that these Langerhans' cells are essential in the development of the contact dermatitis reaction. Over the next ten years it may well become possible to learn how to paralyze this system temporarily and prevent reactions to certain substances, or to test the Langerhans' cells in a biopsy, and predict whether or not their owner is particularly at risk if he handles a certain material.

An interesting observation made very recently is that exposure to ultraviolet light similar to natural sunlight temporarily upsets the normal working of the Langerhans' cells. This may point to a very simple method of regulating their working. The future of this type of research is bright and at present many distinguished and experienced scientists around the world are working on such problems.

9 QUESTIONS AND ANSWERS

As a skin specialist, I am asked many questions about dermatitis – everything from normal anxieties to old wives' tales. I hope that in the course of the book I have been able to allay most fears about the disease as well as dispelling the old wives' tales. For quick and easy reference I have collected here some of the questions I am more commonly asked and have given brief answers.

What is dermatitis?

Quite literally, inflammation of the skin accompanied in most cases by intense itchiness. If untreated, the condition worsens in the following way:

1. The inflamed skin becomes swollen, usually developing tiny blisters which eventually burst and weep.
2. When these dry, a crust forms over the area.
3. In the last stage the skin thickens, with the outer layer constantly flaking off as scales.

The earlier you see your doctor, the more likely your dermatitis can be brought under control.

What's the difference between dermatitis and eczema?

They are the same disease. Eczema is the popular word for the atopic dermatitis which affects mainly children, though all ages can suffer from it. Dermatitis is the preferred medical word.

How common is dermatitis?

It is difficult to give a quick and simple answer to this question. In childhood up to 10 per cent of the under-fives may have atopic dermatitis. In school children the numbers affected appear to be much lower. In adult life the pattern changes, so while atopic dermatitis is much less common, contact dermatitis becomes more frequent. There are variations depending on type of employment and part of the world, but in broad terms it can be said that dermatitis is by far the commonest skin condition the world over.

Does stress bring it on?
In short, sometimes. What is stress for one person is normal life for another, but periods of bereavement, anxiety over job prospects and, for teenagers, examinations can all be associated with either the development of dermatitis for the first time, or a flare up of dermatitis already present.

Is it contagious?
Uncomplicated dermatitis is not contagious. However, secondary infection may be passed on to those who come into close contact, and it is therefore important to see your doctor if you develop infected lesions.

Will it spread?
Some forms of dermatitis such as neurodermatitis remain limited for long periods of time to small areas of skin. In other types, the dermatitis spreads rapidly and may involve extensive areas of the body. Sensible and prompt treatment will in almost all cases prevent or at least reduce spread.

What can I do during or after pregnancy to help lessen the risk of my child having dermatitis?
Unless you and your partner both have personal and family histories of atopic dermatitis, your child is no more at risk than any other, even if you already have a child with dermatitis. There is no specific diet or treatment at present which is recognized as being of value, but smoking during pregnancy may be related to a greater risk of your baby developing atopic dermatitis and is not to be encouraged, both for this and also many other reasons. Current evidence would suggest that breast feeding may help prevent dermatitis in some cases and it is therefore advisable to plan to breast feed your child if at all possible.

Are cortisone-containing creams safe for my child?
Doctors are concerned about the possibility of side-effects from cortisone creams but these are very rare and are generally far outweighed by the benefit these creams can bring about if sensibly used. By sensible I mean:

1. Use only the cream prescribed for your child, not the one prescribed for any other family member.

2. Be quite sure which cream your doctor wants you to use on your child's face and which on other areas of the body. In general, milder preparations are prescribed for the face than for elsewhere. Do not mix them up.

3. Ask your doctor for exact guidelines about how often to apply these preparations and exactly how much to use at each treatment.

4. Remember that if your child has dry skin, the use of emollients and moisture-retaining preparations will reduce the amount of cortisone creams your child requires.

How quickly does treatment for dermatitis work?

If properly applied, treatment will start to have an effect on your dermatitis within forty-eight hours. As a rule of thumb, it is common to find great improvement in the first two to three weeks of treatment, and after this a gradual slowing up in the improvement; the last little bit is always the slowest.

Can dermatitis be cured?

Frequently the answer is 'yes'. Atopic dermatitis very often clears of its own accord in the first ten years of life. With allergic contact dermatitis identification and avoidance of the material that causes it will quickly result in cure. In other cases improvement can confidently be expected and cure is possible.

Should I join a self-help organization for dermatitis sufferers?

The short answer is 'yes' (if there is one in your country). These organizations differ from country to country but are usually composed of patients, parents and friends of dermatitis sufferers. Most have many local branches which meet several times a year. The meetings often involve a talk from an invited skin specialist from the local hospital, and you will find the other members tremendously friendly and supportive. If you are not already a member why not go along to the next meeting of your local branch and ask the secretary for more details? A list of useful addresses has been included opposite.

USEFUL ADDRESSES

The following organizations should be able to tell you where to get help.

UNITED STATES

The American Academy of Dermatology
1567 Maple Avenue
Evanston, Illinois 60201

The Noah Worcester Dermatological Society
3300 Webster Street
Suite 509
Oakland, California 94609

The Society for Investigative Dermatology
Department of Dermatology
North Carolina Memorial Hospital
Chapel Hill, North Carolina 27514

The Society for Pediatric Dermatology
4200 E. Ninth Avenue, B–153
Denver, Colorado 80262

For advice on soya protein milk:

The American Soybean Association
777 Craig Road
PO Box 27300
St Louis, Missouri 63141

GREAT BRITAIN & EIRE

The National Eczema Society
Tavistock House North
Tavistock Square
London WC1H 9SR

Area contacts:

NORTHERN IRELAND
Mrs M. Paige
33 Garnerville Drive
Belfast BT4 2NZ

EIRE
Mrs V. Bresnihan
5 Woodbine Road
Blackrock
County Dublin

For pure cotton children's clothes

Cotton On
Bankside House
Great Plumpton
Kirkham
Lancashire

CANADA

Canadian Dermatological Association
11 Côte Pedu Palais
Quebec City, Quebec
G1R 2J6
Tel: (418) 694–5200

AUSTRALIA

Australasian College of Dermatologists
271 Bridge Road
Glebe, Sydney
NSW 2037

SOUTH AFRICA

Dermatological Society of South Africa
200 North Park Centre
Corner of 3rd and 7th Avenue
Parktown North
South Africa 2193

INTERNATIONAL DRUG NAME EQUIVALENTS

Generic names (in alphabetical order)	UK trade names	US trade names
acetylated wool alcohols + liquid paraffin	Oilatum	no equivalent found
beclomethasone dipropionate	Propaderm	not available as topical preparation
betamethasone valerate	Betnovate	Valisone
chlorpheniramine maleate	Piriton	Chlor-Trimeton
clobetasol propionate	Dermovate	not available
clobetasone butyrate	Eumovate	not available
fluocinolone acetonide (0.025%)	Synalar	Synalar; Fluonid
fluocinolone acetonide (0.2%)	Synalar Forte	Synalar-HP
flurandrenolone/ flurandenolide (US)	Haelan	Cordran
hydrocortisone	Efcortelan; Hydrocortone; Cortril; etc	Cortril; Alphaderm; Dermacort; etc
hydrocortisone butyrate	Locoid	not available
neomycin sulphate	Nivemycin; Myciguent	not available on its own as topical preparation
oat fraction + liquid paraffin	Aveeno (oilated)	Aveeno (oilated)
promethazine hydrochloride	Phenergan	Phenergan; Remsed
trimeprazine tartrate	Vallergan	Temaril

Generic names (in alphabetical order)	Canadian trade names	Australian trade names	South African trade names
acetylated wool alcohols + liquid paraffin	Oilatum (available as a soap only)	Oilatum Emollient	Oilatum
beclomethasone dipropionate	Propaderm	not available as topical preparation	Propaderm
betamethasone valerate	Betnovate; Betacort; etc	Betnovate; Celestone-V	Betnovate; Persivate; Celestoderm-V
chlorpheniramine maleate	Chlorphen; Novopheniram	Piriton; Chloramin; etc	Chlortrimeton
clobetasol propionate	Dermovate	not available	Dermovate
clobetasone butyrate	Eumovate	Eumovate	Eumovate
fluocinolone acetonide (0.025%)	Synalar; Fluoderm; etc	Synalar	Synalar; Cortoderm
fluocinolone acetonide (0.2%)	Synalar High Potency	Synalar Forte	not available
flurandrenolone/ flurandenolide (Canada)	Drenison	Haelan (discontinued)	not available
hydrocortisone	Cortate; Cortef; etc	Egocort	Procutan
hydrocortisone butyrate	not available	Locoid	Locoid
neomycin sulphate	Myciguent	Myciguent; Siguent Neomycin	not available on its own as topical preparation
oat fraction/ colloidal oatmeal (Canada) + liquid paraffin	Aveeno oilated	Aveeno oilated	no equivalent found
promethazine hydrochloride	Phenergan	Phenergan; Prothazine	Phenergan; Lenazine
trimeprazine tartrate	Panectyl	Vallergan	Vallergan

ACKNOWLEDGEMENTS

The publishers thank the following individuals and organizations for their permission to reproduce photographs. Art Directors Photo Library, London (page 22); Bavaria Verlag, Munich (page 30); Mr I. McKie, Medical Photographer, Department of Dermatology, Glasgow University (pages 13, 27, 38, 39, 42, 49, 51, 62, 63, 67 and 91); the Photographers' Library, London (page 31); NFB Photothèque, Ottawa (page 40); Pictor International, London (page 76); the Welsh National School of Medicine's Department of Medical Illustration (pages 58 and 59); and Zefa, London (pages 29, 32 and 41).

The photographs on the cover and pages 23, 24, 47, 54, 64, 74, 78, 79, 80, 82 and 87 were taken by Dave Brown and Dave Robinson. Most of the modelling for these was done by Elayne Lawrence and Samantha Mortner.

The diagrams on pages 11, 15, 17, 19, 52 and 99 were drawn by David Gifford.

Finally, thanks are due to Jennifer Eaton, BSc, MSc, MPS, for information on international drug name equivalents.

INDEX

Other books in the
Positive Health Guide
Series

ASTHMA AND
HAYFEVER
Dr Allan Knight
Breathing difficulties or a
streaming nose afflict
thousands every year. An
expert allergist explains what
is happening to you and what
you can do to ease the
problem.

PSORIASIS
Prof Ronald Marks
An essential book for
psoriasis sufferers, their
families and all those with a
professional interest in the
condition.

MIGRAINE AND
HEADACHES
Dr Marcia Wilkinson
An eminent migraine clinic
director shows how to avoid
and control the pain.

HIGH BLOOD PRESSURE
**Dr Eoin O'Brien and
Prof Kevin O'Malley**
A comprehensive and
practical guide to detecting,
preventing and controlling
one of the greatest risks to
health and life expectancy.

THE HIGH-FIBRE
COOKBOOK
Pamela Westland
Introduced by
Dr Denis Burkitt
Over 200 delicious, tried and
tested high-fibre dishes to
help you eat well and stay
healthy. Each recipe is
accompanied by calorie, fibre
and fat values.

THE DIABETICS'
DIET BOOK
**Dr Jim Mann and the
Oxford Dietetic Group**
The first book for diabetics
and their dietitians that
shows how to change to the
new high carbohydrate and
fibre diet now recommended
by leading diabetic
organizations around the
world. Features over 140
mouthwatering recipes with
full nutritional analyses.

OVERCOMING
ARTHRITIS
Dr Frank Dudley Hart
A guide to coping with stiff
or aching joints, written by a
leading rheumatologist.

DIABETES
Dr James Anderson
A complete new guide to
healthy living for diabetics,
featuring the recently
developed high carbohydrate
and fibre (HCF) diet
programme.